Cleanliness Throughout Life

Cleanliness Throughout Life

Matthew Petchinsky

Cleanliness Throughout Life: A Guide to Lifelong Hygiene, Health, and Dignity

By: Matthew Petchinsky

Introduction: The Lifelong Power of Cleanliness

Cleanliness is often framed as a routine chore—something to cross off the daily to-do list. But when we take a deeper look, personal hygiene, particularly the act of showering, emerges as far more than a surface-level task. It is a vital practice that underpins our health, influences our self-image, and shapes our experience in the world. Cleanliness is not just a behavior—it is a reflection of how we value ourselves and how we participate in society.

This book, *Cleanliness Throughout Life: A Guide to Lifelong Hygiene, Health, and Dignity*, invites you to rethink personal hygiene through a lifelong lens. From the gentle care routines of infancy to the assisted hygiene needs of old age, the act of staying clean is a dynamic journey that evolves with our bodies, lifestyles, and societal roles. Each life stage brings its own set of challenges and responsibilities, and understanding how hygiene adapts across time can empower us to care for ourselves—and others—more effectively.

At its core, cleanliness is a gateway to physical health. It helps prevent the spread of disease, protects sensitive organs like the skin and mouth, and serves as our first defense against harmful bacteria, viruses, and fungi. From washing hands to bathing the body, these actions support a robust immune system and reduce our exposure to illness.

Yet the power of cleanliness does not stop at the physical. Hygiene has a profound impact on our mental and emotional well-being. Cleanliness is often tied to self-esteem, confidence, and even mood regulation. A person struggling with mental health challenges may neglect hygiene—not out of laziness, but as a symptom of depression, anxiety, or trauma. Conversely, the act of showering, brushing one's teeth, or applying lotion can serve as grounding rituals that promote mental clarity and emotional resilience.

Cleanliness also carries deep social and cultural meaning. In many societies, being clean is seen as a sign of respect—not only for oneself, but for others. It enhances how we are perceived in public spaces, influences job opportunities, and fosters more meaningful social interactions. Poor hygiene can isolate us; good hygiene can empower us.

This book is not just about staying clean—it is about reclaiming hygiene as a tool for lifelong empowerment. Each chapter will guide you through the unique hygiene needs, best practices, and challenges that arise during the various stages of life:

- **In childhood**, hygiene routines become a learning ground for discipline and self-respect.
- **In the teenage years**, hormonal changes and social pressures make hygiene a cornerstone of self-confidence.
- **In adulthood**, it becomes a balancing act between responsibility, time management, and health.
- **In elderhood**, it evolves again—requiring gentleness, support, and a preservation of dignity.

Beyond these stages, we'll explore the **social, cultural, environmental, and technological** influences on cleanliness. We'll examine what it means to live clean in a polluted world, how hygiene intersects with mental health, and how to build supportive systems for those who need help maintaining their routines.

Whether you are a parent trying to teach your child to bathe, a teenager struggling with acne and identity, an overworked adult seeking balance, or a caregiver tending to a senior loved one—this book is your comprehensive guide. More than a manual, it is a celebration of the dignity and vitality that cleanliness brings to our lives.

Cleanliness is not just about scrubbing the surface. It is about renewal. It is about care. It is about showing up for yourself—every day, in every season of life.

Let us begin the journey.

Chapter 1: The Science of Clean—What Hygiene Really Means

Cleanliness is more than just a routine. It is a science, a discipline, and a conscious act of care. In this chapter, we uncover what hygiene truly means in modern life—not just as a health safeguard, but as a powerful expression of respect for ourselves, others, and the environments we inhabit.

Defining Personal Hygiene in Modern Terms

Personal hygiene is defined as a series of daily practices designed to maintain bodily cleanliness, prevent the spread of disease, and preserve physical, mental, and social well-being. In modern terms, personal hygiene encompasses both visible cleanliness (such as a fresh appearance or clean clothing) and invisible maintenance (such as the prevention of bacterial buildup on the skin or in the mouth).

Today, personal hygiene also includes environmental awareness and the intelligent use of technology and sustainable products. The rise of eco-friendly soaps, biodegradable hygiene tools, and smart toothbrushes shows that hygiene is no longer just about function—it's about mindfulness and ethics, too. We are no longer just cleaning ourselves; we are consciously managing the ecosystems of our bodies and homes.

Hygiene is also culturally contextual. What's considered "clean" may vary between societies, but the core principles remain constant: remove waste, reduce odor, eliminate harmful microbes, and maintain health.

Above all, hygiene today is personal. It must be tailored to one's age, skin type, health conditions, cultural needs, and lifestyle. It is no longer a one-size-fits-all checklist—it is a dynamic, adaptive process that evolves as we do.

Key Hygiene Areas: Skin, Teeth, Hands, Hair, Nails, and Body Functions

Let's break down the six primary zones of personal hygiene and understand their importance:

1. Skin Hygiene

The skin is our body's largest organ and first line of defense. It absorbs toxins, regulates temperature, and acts as a shield against bacteria. Regular bathing or showering removes sweat, dead skin cells, dirt, allergens, and pathogens that accumulate throughout the day. Moisturizing after bathing preserves the skin barrier, preventing cracking, dryness, and infection.

Proper skin hygiene also includes:

- Using products suited to your skin type (oily, dry, sensitive, etc.)
- Gentle exfoliation (once or twice a week) to avoid buildup
- Wearing breathable clothing and regularly washing garments

2. Oral Hygiene (Teeth and Mouth)

Dental hygiene is essential for digestion, confidence, and disease prevention. Brushing twice daily, flossing, and rinsing with mouthwash reduce the buildup of plaque, which can lead to tooth decay, gum disease, bad breath, and even heart disease.

Key oral practices:

- Use fluoride toothpaste to strengthen enamel
- Replace toothbrushes every 3 months
- Visit the dentist at least once a year
- Scrub or clean the tongue to remove bacteria

3. Hand Hygiene

Hands are the most common vehicles for transmitting germs. Proper handwashing is one of the most effective tools in stopping the spread of illnesses—from colds and flu to more serious viruses and gastrointestinal diseases.

Effective hand hygiene includes:

- Washing with soap and water for 20 seconds
- Using hand sanitizer when soap isn't available
- Cleaning under fingernails and between fingers
- Washing hands before meals, after bathroom use, after touching public surfaces, or caring for someone sick

4. Hair Hygiene

Scalp and hair health affect everything from personal appearance to comfort. Dirty or unwashed hair can attract parasites (like lice), cause scalp infections, and become a source of odor. Oily build-up can block pores, while overwashing can strip the scalp of its protective oils.

Modern hair hygiene includes:

- Choosing a shampoo that suits your scalp type
- Conditioning regularly for manageability
- Washing frequency based on lifestyle (e.g., more often for athletes or outdoor workers)
- Keeping facial hair trimmed and clean

5. Nail Hygiene

Fingernails and toenails can harbor dirt, bacteria, and fungi, especially in the crevices. Long or unclean nails can cause infection or injury. Key practices:

- Keep nails trimmed and filed
- Clean under nails daily
- Avoid biting nails, which introduces germs to the mouth
- Disinfect tools used for grooming

6. Body Function Hygiene

Maintaining cleanliness in areas associated with elimination and reproduction is essential for health, comfort, and confidence. This includes:

- Regular washing of genital areas with water and gentle, fragrance-free products
- Safe and clean menstrual product usage
- Managing sweat with breathable fabrics and deodorants
- Wiping front to back to prevent infection (especially important for women)
- Addressing incontinence with proper products and routines

The Link Between Hygiene and Disease Prevention

Scientific studies have repeatedly confirmed the powerful link between personal hygiene and public health. Hand hygiene alone can reduce respiratory illness by 16–21% and diarrheal disease by up to 40%. Cleanliness interrupts the transmission of harmful microorganisms that thrive in sweat, dirt, and bodily secretions.

Some examples of hygiene-preventable illnesses include:

- Influenza and common colds
- COVID-19
- Foodborne illnesses (like salmonella and norovirus)
- Fungal infections (like athlete's foot)
- Dental diseases (gingivitis, cavities)
- Skin conditions (eczema, acne, bacterial rashes)

Moreover, hospital and eldercare environments heavily rely on hygiene to prevent the spread of antibiotic-resistant superbugs. In this sense, personal hygiene is not just self-care—it is disease control and a public health duty.

Hygiene as an Act of Self-Respect and Self-Love

Cleanliness isn't just about avoiding illness—it's about how we feel in our bodies. Showering after a long day, washing our faces in the morning, or combing our hair before an interview are small rituals of respect that say: *I am worth caring for.*

Maintaining hygiene:

- Boosts **confidence** and **self-image**
- Reinforces **boundaries** and **autonomy** over one's body
- Creates a foundation for **mental stability** through daily structure
- Reflects **personal values**, such as discipline, attention to detail, and pride

For those who struggle with mental health, chronic illness, or disability, even simple hygiene acts can feel monumental. But when accomplished—even in small ways—they can help rebuild a sense of agency and dignity.

Self-respect through hygiene doesn't mean perfection. It means consistency, adaptability, and the courage to show up for ourselves—again and again.

In Summary

Personal hygiene is the science and art of staying clean in a complex world. It touches every part of our lives—our health, emotions, relationships, and even how we engage with our communities. As this chapter has shown, hygiene is a personal revolution. It's a daily opportunity to show up for ourselves with care, presence, and pride.

Regardless of where you are on that journey, the foundation of clean living starts here.

Chapter 2: Ancient Baths to Antibacterial Soaps—A History of Hygiene

To understand the importance of personal hygiene in the modern world, we must first look back. The journey of cleanliness spans thousands of years, shaped by culture, science, religion, war, and survival. Hygiene has not always been a personal or private matter—it has often been deeply public, spiritual, and even political. This chapter explores the evolution of hygiene practices, from the grand public baths of antiquity to the era of antibacterial soaps and hygiene apps, revealing how our understanding of cleanliness has changed over time—and what it means for us today.

Hygiene Practices in Ancient Civilizations

Long before hand sanitizers and toothpaste, ancient civilizations had already developed advanced and meaningful hygiene systems. Cleanliness was often tied to spiritual purity, social standing, and health—even if the scientific understanding of germs didn't yet exist.

1. Ancient Egypt

Egyptians viewed cleanliness as a sacred duty. Bathing multiple times a day was common, especially among the wealthy. They used **natron salts, alabaster jars of perfumed oils**, and **early soaps made from animal fat and clay** to clean the body. Shaving body hair was also practiced for hygiene and religious reasons.

Priests were expected to be exceptionally clean, often shaving their entire bodies and washing up to four times a day to serve the gods. Hygiene in Egypt wasn't just routine—it was ritual.

2. Ancient India

The Indus Valley Civilization (as early as 2600 BCE) boasted **remarkably sophisticated sanitation systems**. Archaeological findings show homes with private bathing areas and an extensive drainage system that carried waste away from cities.

In later periods, **Ayurveda**—India's traditional medicine—emphasized hygiene as vital to health, with daily rituals like *dinacharya* (morning cleansing routines), oil pulling, and herbal bathing as foundations for balance in body and spirit.

3. Ancient Rome and Greece

The Romans may be the most iconic ancient hygienists. Their cities featured sprawling **public bathhouses (thermae)**, which were social hubs as well as cleansing stations. Citizens would cycle through warm (tepidarium), hot (caldarium), and cold (frigidarium) rooms, scrubbing themselves with oils and scraping off sweat and dirt using a tool called a *strigil*.

Greek physicians like **Hippocrates** also emphasized the link between hygiene and disease prevention, even without the modern concept of germs. Cleanliness was seen as a preventative health measure and a sign of moral virtue.

4. Ancient China

Chinese hygiene traditions were deeply rooted in **Confucian and Taoist** philosophies. While public bathhouses were also common, cleanliness extended to clothing rituals, nail grooming, and dental practices. The use of **green tea and herbal rinses** for oral health was a standard practice, and hygiene was associated with inner harmony and respect for others.

Across these cultures, we see a recurring theme: **cleanliness equals respect**—for oneself, for others, and for the divine.

The Decline of Cleanliness in the Middle Ages

After the fall of the Roman Empire, much of Europe's public sanitation infrastructure crumbled. The communal bathhouses fell into disrepair, and with them, the widespread practice of routine bathing. This was not just due to a lack of resources—it was also philosophical and religious.

1. Misconceptions and Fear

In medieval Europe, it was commonly believed that **bathing opened the pores and made the body vulnerable to disease**, especially during plague outbreaks. Water, once seen as purifying, was now feared. Many people turned to **dry hygiene**, such as wiping the skin with cloths and changing undergarments as substitutes for bathing.

2. The Church's Influence

The rise of Christian asceticism also contributed to the decline of bathing. Cleanliness was increasingly seen as vanity or even sinful indulgence. While some monastic communities maintained hygiene rituals, public bathing was discouraged and often associated with immoral behavior or prostitution.

3. The Black Death and Urban Filth

By the 14th century, Europe was ravaged by the Black Death. Streets ran with waste, chamber pots were dumped into rivers, and cities reeked of unwashed bodies. Although people recognized that filth brought disease, the **miasma theory** (bad air causing illness) still dominated. There was no real understanding of bacteria, viruses, or contagion via touch—only that foul odors meant danger.

In contrast, Islamic and Asian regions maintained better hygiene practices during this time. In Islamic cultures, **ritual washing (wudu)** before prayer and personal cleanliness remained vital, preserving ancient traditions that Europe had largely abandoned.

Renaissance Revival and the Rise of Sanitation Science

The Renaissance was not just a rebirth of art and philosophy—it was a slow rediscovery of cleanliness.

1. The Return of Bathing

In the 16th and 17th centuries, European elites slowly began embracing bathing again, although it remained more of a luxury than a daily necessity. **Perfume and powdered wigs** were used to mask body odor, and washing with cloths remained more common than full immersion in water.

2. Enlightenment and Early Science

The 18th century brought forward thinkers like **Antonie van Leeuwenhoek**, who used microscopes to observe microorganisms. Though germ theory hadn't yet been developed, curiosity about invisible agents of illness began to take root.

Soap-making also became more sophisticated during this time. Soap shifted from a homemade necessity to a commercial product, especially in regions like France and Italy, where perfumed soaps became symbols of refinement.

3. The Sanitary Revolution

The true shift came in the 19th century, with the rise of **modern public health movements**. Two events were pivotal:

- **John Snow's 1854 cholera investigation** in London, which linked water contamination to disease.
- **Louis Pasteur's germ theory**, which proved that microorganisms cause illness.

These discoveries revolutionized hygiene. Cities began building sewer systems, promoting clean drinking water, and investing in public health education. Hospitals embraced handwashing. Soap became a household staple. The concept of "being clean to stay healthy" was now a scientifically validated truth.

20th–21st Century Revolutions in Hygiene

With the dawn of the modern era, hygiene practices became deeply embedded in daily life—and expanded in scope and innovation.

1. The Hygiene Boom

By the early 20th century, mass-produced soap, toothpaste, deodorant, and sanitary products became affordable and accessible. Public health campaigns promoted regular handwashing, dental care, and vaccinations. Schools taught hygiene as part of education, and military organizations emphasized cleanliness to prevent outbreaks.

Hygiene was no longer just a personal matter—it became **a national goal** tied to productivity, morality, and patriotism.

2. Antibacterial Obsession

In the late 20th century, the rise of **antibacterial soaps, hand sanitizers, and antiseptics** created a cultural obsession with killing germs. While this helped reduce some infections, overuse has contributed to **antibiotic resistance** and disrupted natural skin microbiomes.

At the same time, better access to plumbing and electricity made daily bathing normal in many parts of the world. Cleanliness became a **standard of living**, and poor hygiene was often seen (sometimes unfairly) as a sign of poverty or neglect.

3. Digital Hygiene and Innovation

Today, we are entering an era of **technological hygiene**:

- Smart toothbrushes track brushing habits
- AI-powered skincare apps recommend personalized regimens
- Water-saving shower heads reduce waste
- Wearable devices monitor sweat and odor levels
- Eco-friendly hygiene products help us clean without polluting

During the COVID-19 pandemic, the world was reminded of the life-saving power of basic hygiene. Handwashing, surface sanitizing, and cough etiquette became top priorities globally—reinforcing that the lessons of the past remain urgent today.

In Summary

The story of hygiene is the story of civilization. From the sacred cleansing rituals of ancient Egypt to the gleaming dental tools of modern dentistry, from communal Roman baths to personalized hygiene apps, our cleanliness practices have always reflected what we believe about the body, health, and society.

Understanding this history helps us make better choices today. It reminds us that hygiene is not just reactive—it is **preventative, proactive, and deeply personal**. It connects us to generations before us and lays a foundation for the health and dignity of those who follow.

Chapter 3: Childhood Clean—Building Healthy Habits from Day One

Childhood is the most formative period in a person's life, not only in terms of physical and emotional development but also in the formation of lifelong habits. Among the most important of these habits is personal hygiene. Teaching children the value of cleanliness isn't simply about keeping them free from germs—it's about empowering them with a framework for self-care, health, confidence, and respect for others.

In this chapter, we explore how to make hygiene fun, effective, and meaningful for children, while also addressing the common struggles many families face when building these essential routines.

Teaching Kids About Hygiene Through Routines and Play

Children learn best through **structure, repetition, and play**. Unlike adults who may respond to logical reasoning or personal motivation, young children thrive on interactive learning and routine-based guidance. When hygiene is taught consistently and framed as an enjoyable activity, it becomes second nature over time.

1. Daily Routines as Learning Foundations

Routine creates security for children. Set hygiene tasks at predictable times (e.g., brushing teeth after breakfast and before bed, bathing after dinner) to give them structure. Eventually, these rituals become embedded in their sense of normalcy.

Examples:

- **Morning Hygiene Routine:** Brush teeth, wash face, comb hair, change into clean clothes
- **Evening Routine:** Bath or shower, brush teeth, put on pajamas, wash hands before bedtime snack or story

2. Hygiene Through Play

Play-based learning makes hygiene approachable and engaging.
Creative methods include:

- **Bath time games** (toy boats, waterproof storybooks)
- **"Germ monster" storytelling** to explain invisible dirt
- **Hygiene songs and rhymes** for brushing and handwashing ("This is the way we brush our teeth...")
- **Sticker charts and reward systems** for completing daily hygiene tasks
- **Pretend play** with dolls or action figures modeling cleanliness behaviors

This combination of ritual and imagination helps children associate hygiene with fun, not frustration.

Addressing Common Resistance: Bath Refusal, Teeth Brushing, and More

Many parents face resistance when introducing hygiene habits, especially during toddlerhood and early school years. This resistance is normal but can be overcome with empathy, patience, and strategy.

1. Bath Time Battles

Children may resist bathing for reasons such as fear of water, dislike of shampoo in the eyes, or simply not wanting to interrupt playtime.

Solutions:

- Use **tear-free shampoo** and **soft washcloths**
- Play calming music or let them choose a **bathtime playlist**
- Offer **bath crayons**, waterproof toys, or bubbles
- Let the child help fill the tub or choose the towel
- Create a **story or adventure** (e.g., "We're swimming through space!")

2. Tooth Brushing Challenges

Brushing teeth can feel invasive or boring to a child. Some kids dislike the taste of toothpaste or don't understand the purpose.

Solutions:

- Use **flavored or fun-colored toothpaste**
- Let them pick their **toothbrush design** (e.g., with characters they love)
- Brush **together**—modeling builds trust
- Use **apps or timers** that make brushing a mini-game
- Reward with stickers or a fun storytime after brushing

3. Resistance to Hair Grooming or Nail Trimming

Tangles and tender scalps often cause children to fear brushing, and nail cutting can feel scary.

Solutions:

- Use **detangling spray** and **wide-tooth combs**
- Trim nails during nap time or after a warm bath
- Let them see you trim your nails first to reduce fear
- Give them a **grooming toy set** so they can "practice" on dolls

4. Forgetting to Wash Hands or Wipe Properly

These tasks require reminders, especially when children are transitioning to independence.

Solutions:

- Hang **visual charts** by the sink and toilet
- Use **color-changing soaps** or fun-smelling handwash
- Reward proper hygiene with praise or fun stamps
- Use **educational videos or books** that show other children modeling good habits

The key is to shift hygiene from a **battle of wills** to a **shared adventure**, where the child feels safe, capable, and praised.

Parental Modeling and Hygiene Education Tools

Children mirror what they see. A child who sees caregivers neglect their own hygiene is unlikely to value it. On the other hand, a parent who models cleanliness with warmth and consistency creates a silent but powerful lesson.

1. Be the Example

- Let your child see you brushing your teeth or washing your face.
- Narrate your own hygiene choices ("I'm washing my hands after using the bathroom to keep germs away").
- Maintain your own grooming so the standard is visible and lived.

2. Involve Children in Decision-Making
Children love autonomy. Involve them by:

- Letting them pick soap or shampoo at the store
- Choosing the toothbrush or bath towel
- Helping prepare a "toothbrush station" or hygiene kit

3. Use Media and Learning Tools
There are many educational tools available to support hygiene teaching:

- **YouTube videos and cartoons** about hygiene (age-appropriate)
- **Children's books** with characters who model clean habits
- **Educational apps** that turn brushing or handwashing into games
- **Printable hygiene trackers** with stars or coloring boxes

Make hygiene part of your child's world—not just a chore, but a value.

Childhood Hygiene Checklists and Fun Reinforcement

Children thrive on visual and tactile feedback. Having a hygiene checklist gives them a sense of responsibility, completion, and reward.

Daily Hygiene Checklist (Ages 3–7)

- Brush teeth (morning and night)
- Wash hands (after toilet, before eating)
- Comb or brush hair
- Wipe properly after bathroom use
- Wear clean clothes and socks
- Take a bath/shower (at least every other day)
- Trim nails weekly (with help)

Fun Reinforcement Ideas

- **Sticker charts** that lead to a weekly reward
- **"Hygiene Hero" badges** or certificates
- **Treasure boxes** for completing routines
- **Story time only after "clean" checklist is complete**
- Let them "teach" a stuffed animal or doll how to brush or bathe

The goal is not perfection—it's **consistency, pride, and participation**.

In Summary

Cleanliness in childhood is not about scrubbing every inch of skin. It's about instilling values, building rituals, and helping children feel empowered to care for their bodies. A child who learns to brush their teeth or wash their hands is learning far more than hygiene—they are learning **responsibility, self-worth, and discipline**.

By turning hygiene into a shared experience filled with play, encouragement, and love, parents lay the foundation for healthy habits that can last a lifetime. And when a child learns to care for their body from day one, they step into adulthood with tools that benefit every area of their life.

Chapter 4: Teenage Hygiene—Navigating Puberty and Self-Image

The teenage years are a time of profound change. Bodies transform, emotions intensify, and identities begin to take shape. In this chapter of life, hygiene becomes far more than a routine—it becomes a **survival skill** and a **tool for self-definition**.

Puberty introduces a host of new physical processes, from sweat and skin changes to menstrual cycles and facial hair growth. These biological shifts demand more advanced, attentive, and frequent hygiene practices. However, navigating these needs is often complicated by emotional turbulence, self-consciousness, and fluctuating confidence.

This chapter addresses the practical, emotional, and psychological aspects of hygiene during adolescence and offers real-world strategies to help teens take ownership of their health and identity.

Hormonal Changes and Increased Hygiene Needs

Puberty is driven by hormones—chemical messengers that trigger growth and change. Estrogen, testosterone, and other hormones begin influencing the body's development in dramatic ways, affecting not only the reproductive system but also the skin, hair, sweat glands, and mood.

1. Increased Sweat and Sebum Production

Teenagers experience a surge in activity from sebaceous (oil) glands and sweat glands, especially in the armpits, groin, and face. These changes result in:

- **Oily skin**
- **Greasy hair**
- **Stronger body odor**

Daily showers, especially after physical activity, become more important during this stage. Antiperspirants and deodorants may also be introduced for the first time.

2. Growth of Body Hair

Hair begins to grow in new places—underarms, legs, arms, face (in boys), and the pubic region. This requires decisions about grooming, shaving, and personal comfort.

3. Menstruation

For girls, the onset of periods is a major milestone. It introduces the need for **menstrual hygiene education**, product use (pads, tampons, menstrual cups), and understanding the emotional and physical fluctuations that accompany hormonal cycles.

Puberty doesn't just increase hygiene needs—it creates entirely **new ones**, all of which must be addressed with sensitivity, clarity, and confidence-building tools.

Acne, Body Odor, Shaving, and Menstrual Care

While each teen's experience is unique, several hygiene concerns are almost universal during puberty. Addressing them with practical solutions and emotional validation is key to building good lifelong habits.

1. Acne and Skin Care

Acne is caused by clogged pores due to oil, dead skin cells, and bacteria. Teens often experience:

- Whiteheads, blackheads, and pimples
- Inflammation or cystic acne in severe cases

Hygiene Strategies:

- Use a gentle **non-comedogenic cleanser** twice a day
- Avoid over-washing, which can irritate the skin
- Never pop pimples—this can worsen inflammation and cause scarring
- Use **oil-free moisturizers** and **SPF** daily
- In serious cases, consult a dermatologist for treatment options

2. Body Odor and Sweat Control

Bacteria feeding on sweat causes body odor, especially in the armpits and feet. Teens should:

- Shower daily, especially after exercise
- Change clothes (especially underwear and socks) daily
- Use **aluminum-free deodorant** or antiperspirants depending on preference
- Wash shoes and use foot powder for odor control if necessary

3. Shaving and Hair Grooming

Shaving is a personal choice influenced by comfort, culture, and social expectations.

Tips for Beginners:

- Use **clean, sharp razors** and shave in the direction of hair growth
- Apply warm water to soften hair and prevent irritation
- Use gentle **shaving creams or gels**
- Consider electric shavers for ease and safety
- Moisturize afterward to prevent razor burn

4. Menstrual Care

For menstruating teens, hygiene becomes a monthly priority.

Hygiene Guidelines:

- Change pads or tampons every 4–6 hours
- Wash hands before and after handling menstrual products
- Rinse or shower daily during menstruation to feel fresh
- Use unscented, pH-balanced intimate washes (or just water)
- Track cycles to prepare ahead and avoid surprises

Offering young people a **judgment-free space** to ask questions and make their own hygiene decisions is critical. Provide options, education, and support—never shame.

Mental Health and Hygiene During Identity Formation

Adolescence is not just about physical transformation—it's also the **age of identity exploration**. Teens begin to ask: *Who am I? How do others see me? Am I normal?* These questions can create anxiety, self-doubt, and self-consciousness that deeply affect hygiene routines.

1. Body Image and Self-Esteem

Teens who feel ashamed of acne, body odor, or weight may avoid hygiene tasks out of discouragement or embarrassment. A lack of confidence can lead to hygiene neglect, just as poor hygiene can damage self-image—a feedback loop that must be broken with compassion.

2. Depression and Executive Dysfunction

Mental health struggles often begin in the teen years. Depression, ADHD, anxiety, and trauma can impair a teen's ability to maintain hygiene—not due to laziness, but because of **overwhelm, fatigue, or dissociation**.

Supportive strategies:

- Break hygiene into **micro-tasks** ("Just brush teeth today," "Take a 3-minute shower")
- Use visual schedules or checklists
- Pair hygiene with rewards or calming routines
- Offer emotional support, not criticism
- Consider therapy or counseling for ongoing struggles

3. Social Pressures and Peer Influence

Peers often influence hygiene choices—positively or negatively. A teen may adopt better grooming habits to fit in, or may feel shame due to teasing or bullying.

Helping teens find **their own standards**, instead of blindly chasing trends, builds internal resilience. Reinforce that hygiene is for self-care, not just social approval.

Strategies for Confidence and Independence

Teenagers crave independence—but also need gentle guidance. Hygiene is a perfect opportunity to practice **self-governance, routine-building, and personal responsibility**.

1. Empowerment Through Ownership

- Let teens choose their own products (shampoo, deodorant, razors)
- Allow them privacy during hygiene routines
- Let them personalize their hygiene schedule (morning showers vs. evening)

2. Positive Reinforcement

- Acknowledge improvements ("I see you've been brushing your teeth every day—great job.")
- Compliment their clean appearance, breath, or scent
- Offer incentives like nicer skincare products or time privileges when they meet hygiene goals

3. Use Tools and Technology

- Hygiene reminder apps or calendars
- YouTube tutorials for shaving, skincare, or hair grooming
- Social media accounts that promote body positivity and clean habits

4. Talk About the Why

Help teens understand that hygiene isn't about perfection—it's about **comfort, confidence, health, and dignity**. When teens grasp the personal benefits (fewer pimples, fresher breath, better sleep), they are more likely to stay consistent.

In Summary

Teenage hygiene is not just about physical upkeep—it's a vital part of becoming independent, confident, and healthy. While the body undergoes dramatic changes, hygiene becomes a stabilizing ritual that helps teens feel in control, respected, and presentable.

The teen years may be turbulent, but when young people are empowered with accurate information, emotional support, and real autonomy, hygiene becomes not just a habit—but a declaration of self-worth.

Maintaining hygiene during adulthood is a whole new challenge—and a deeply rewarding one.

Chapter 5: Adult Hygiene—Routines for the Real World

Adulthood is often characterized by complexity—packed schedules, career demands, relationship obligations, parenting responsibilities, financial pressure, and limited personal time. Amid the hustle of daily life, personal hygiene can either serve as a grounding routine or become one of the first things to be neglected.

In this chapter, we explore the unique hygiene challenges and opportunities adults face. We'll look at how lifestyle, diet, relationships, and mental health influence personal care, and offer practical tools to maintain hygiene as a form of efficient self-respect, not just ritual cleanliness.

Hygiene Amidst Busy Schedules, Work, and Relationships

As children and teens, personal hygiene is often monitored and enforced by caregivers. But as adults, the responsibility falls squarely on our shoulders. The shift from external accountability to internal discipline can either empower us—or, during burnout phases, overwhelm us.

1. Time Management and Hygiene

Adults often skip hygiene rituals not due to lack of awareness, but due to exhaustion or packed routines. However, integrating hygiene into your schedule strategically can make it easier and less stressful.

Strategies:

- **Establish predictable rituals** (e.g., shower every morning before work or every night before bed)
- **Pair hygiene with existing habits** (brush teeth while waiting for coffee to brew, apply skincare while watching a favorite show)
- **Batch grooming tasks** (trim nails, shave, or do skincare all on the same day each week)
- **Use the "2-minute rule"**: If it takes under 2 minutes (like flossing), do it immediately

2. Professional Appearance and Hygiene

In most workplaces, hygiene is not just about personal comfort—it's about perception. Cleanliness affects:

- First impressions
- Respect from peers and clients
- Confidence in communication
- Career advancement (consciously or unconsciously)

Maintaining clean clothes, fresh breath, neat hair, and body odor control communicates competence, discipline, and attention to detail.

3. Hygiene and Relationships

Whether dating, cohabitating, parenting, or married, hygiene becomes a shared dynamic. In romantic partnerships, unaddressed hygiene issues can cause resentment, discomfort, and loss of intimacy.

Communication Tips:

- Discuss hygiene openly but respectfully ("I feel closer to you when we both take care of ourselves.")
- Share routines together (e.g., couples' skincare nights)
- Support partners through hygiene struggles due to illness, depression, or postpartum changes

Hygiene in relationships is not just about looking good—it's about showing care, effort, and mutual respect.

Diet, Exercise, and Stress Impact on Cleanliness

Your hygiene needs don't exist in isolation—they're deeply intertwined with how you live.

1. Diet and Hygiene

What you eat affects how your body smells, how your skin behaves, and how your breath is perceived.

Key Diet-Hygiene Links:

- **Garlic, onions, and spicy foods** can increase body odor
- **Sugary foods** promote bad breath and tooth decay
- **Dairy and greasy foods** may exacerbate acne
- **Hydration** helps flush toxins and reduces dry skin or bad breath
- **Fiber-rich foods** improve digestion and reduce odor in bowel movements

Eating clean supports staying clean.

2. Exercise and Sweat Hygiene

Exercise promotes circulation, skin health, mood stability, and physical fitness—but it also increases sweat, oil production, and odor.

Post-workout Hygiene Tips:

- Shower as soon as possible after intense activity
- Wash gym clothes after every use
- Keep deodorant, wipes, or a change of clothes in your gym bag
- Clean your gear—yoga mats, headphones, and water bottles

Don't let sweat settle—your skin and self-esteem will thank you.

3. Stress and Hygiene Breakdown

Chronic stress affects everything—sleep patterns, appetite, libido, skin, and hygiene motivation. Under stress, it's common to:

- Skip showers
- Sleep in unwashed clothes
- Forget to brush teeth or hair
- Stop doing laundry
- Avoid social grooming tasks (shaving, skincare)

Recognizing stress as a hygiene disruptor allows for intervention. Even the act of brushing your teeth or splashing water on your face can help reset your nervous system and signal self-preservation.

Smart Hygiene Habits for Modern Adults

Technology, accessibility, and innovation have made adult hygiene more customizable and convenient than ever. When used mindfully, modern tools can help streamline routines and promote consistency.

1. Hygiene Tech and Tools

- **Electric toothbrushes** with pressure sensors and built-in timers
- **Shower timers or speakers** to create ritual and efficiency
- **Skin analysis apps** that offer personalized skincare advice
- **Subscription boxes** for razors, skincare, or hygiene kits
- **UV toothbrush sanitizers** or reusable face towels

Integrate smart hygiene—not just flashy products, but functional solutions that fit your life.

2. On-the-Go Hygiene Solutions

Busy professionals and parents often need mobile hygiene fixes:

- **Mini hygiene kits** (deodorant, face wipes, floss, cologne/perfume)
- **Portable bidets** or wet wipes for clean restroom experiences
- **Dry shampoo** for quick hair refreshment
- **Hand sanitizer** and breath mints at arm's reach

These tools help maintain freshness and confidence between full routines.

3. Simplifying and Decluttering Routines

You don't need 12 skincare steps or an entire cabinet of products to stay clean. A minimalist approach saves time and money.

Basic daily routine (customizable):

- Shower or wash key areas (underarms, groin, feet)
- Brush teeth and tongue
- Deodorant
- Moisturizer or sunscreen
- Hair grooming

Build from this baseline depending on your goals (e.g., skincare, shaving, beard maintenance).

Self-Care vs. Neglect: The Fine Line

Adults often struggle with knowing when they are practicing self-care versus when they are rationalizing neglect.

1. The Myth of "I'm Too Busy"

Sometimes skipping hygiene feels justified. But repeated neglect sends harmful messages to the subconscious: *I don't matter today.* That's not self-care—that's erosion of self-worth.

Quick questions to assess:

- Am I skipping hygiene because I'm overwhelmed, not because I'm prioritizing joy?
- Is my current state making me feel better or worse?
- Would I treat a loved one this way if they were in my position?

2. Compassionate Hygiene

When energy is low, aim for the **bare minimum self-respect routine**:

- Brush teeth, splash face with water
- Change underwear and socks
- Drink water and apply moisturizer

It's not all-or-nothing. Every act of care—however small—is a message to your body: *You are worth the effort.*

3. Redefining Hygiene as Self-Care

Don't treat hygiene as a punishment or social obligation. Treat it as your **daily reset button**—an opportunity to:

- Reclaim control in chaotic days
- Feel fresh and capable
- Reconnect with your body
- Begin again

Even the most basic hygiene routines can become therapeutic when approached with intention and self-kindness.

In Summary

Adult hygiene is about **adaptability, intentionality, and dignity**. It's the thread that ties together our inner world and outer presence. It evolves with our responsibilities, our relationships, and our understanding of self-worth.

Whether you're managing a career, a household, or your mental health—hygiene doesn't have to be elaborate. It just has to be consistent, personal, and respectful.

Chapter 6: Elder Hygiene—Cleanliness in Later Years

Aging brings with it the quiet yet persistent transformation of the body. Skin becomes fragile, joints ache, reflexes slow, and energy wanes. The simple routines of daily hygiene that were once automatic can become daunting tasks. Yet, even in later life, the need for cleanliness remains—not only as a matter of physical health but also as a vital link to dignity, comfort, and emotional well-being.

This chapter explores the hygiene challenges that arise with aging, the specialized tools and strategies that support elder care, and the powerful connection between hygiene and self-worth in one's later years.

Aging Skin, Arthritis, and Mobility Challenges
As the body ages, physiological changes affect how elders interact with their environment—including how they bathe, groom, and maintain personal hygiene.

1. Skin Changes and Sensitivities
Older adults experience a decrease in **collagen, elastin, and natural oils**, leading to:

- Thinner, more delicate skin prone to tears
- Increased dryness, itching, or flakiness
- Heightened sensitivity to soaps, detergents, and hot water

Hygiene Considerations:

- Use **fragrance-free, moisturizing cleansers**
- Apply **gentle body lotions** after bathing to reduce dryness
- Limit hot showers to avoid stripping natural oils
- Avoid scrubbing too harshly—pat skin dry with soft towels

2. Arthritis and Joint Stiffness

Arthritis, a common condition among elders, affects the hands, hips, knees, and spine, making it difficult to perform even basic grooming tasks like:

- Holding a toothbrush or razor
- Reaching behind the back in the shower
- Trimming nails
- Standing for long periods

Solutions:

- Use **ergonomic tools with wide grips**
- Install **shower chairs**, **grab bars**, and **non-slip mats**
- Allow more time for hygiene routines
- Incorporate **adaptive tools** like long-handled brushes and electric toothbrushes

3. Mobility and Balance Issues

Declining strength and balance make bathing risky. Slips and falls in the bathroom are one of the leading causes of injury in seniors.

Preventative Actions:

- Ensure the bathroom is **well-lit and clutter-free**
- Use **walk-in tubs** or **low-threshold showers**
- Add **raised toilet seats** and **support rails**
- Consider **in-home occupational therapy assessments** for tailored safety adjustments

When physical limitations begin to interfere with hygiene, support systems and adaptive solutions are critical for preserving autonomy and minimizing risk.

Maintaining Dignity While Receiving Hygiene Help

For many elders, needing help with personal hygiene is emotionally difficult. It may trigger feelings of shame, helplessness, or even depression. After a lifetime of independence, relying on someone else for bathing or toileting can feel like a personal loss.

1. Understanding the Emotional Weight

- Hygiene tasks are intimate and private—needing assistance in these areas can be humiliating
- Memory loss or cognitive impairment may cause confusion or resistance during care
- Some elders may fear being a burden to caregivers or family

2. Building Trust and Respect

Caregivers, whether family or professionals, must approach hygiene assistance with **empathy, discretion, and patience.**

Best Practices:

- Always explain what you're doing and why
- Allow the elder to do whatever they can independently
- Use **covering towels or robes** to preserve modesty during sponge baths or changes
- Maintain a **calm, respectful tone**, even if the elder resists help
- Offer **choices** (e.g., "Would you like to shower now or after breakfast?")

Caregivers should remember: the goal is not just cleanliness, but **preservation of identity and dignity.**

Specialized Tools and Products for Elderly Care

Advances in home healthcare and assistive technology have made hygiene safer and more accessible for aging individuals.

1. Bathing Aids

- **Shower chairs** and **transfer benches** to reduce fall risk
- **Handheld showerheads** for better control
- **No-rinse body washes** and **shampoo caps** for bedridden individuals
- **Long-handled scrubbers** for reaching difficult areas
- **Bathing gloves** to help caregivers cleanse skin gently

2. Dental and Oral Hygiene Tools

- **Electric toothbrushes** with large handles for easy grip
- **Water flossers** for those with dexterity issues
- **Mouth moisturizing sprays** for dry mouth caused by medications
- **Denture cleaning tablets and brushes**

Regular dental care is essential in elder years to prevent infections and maintain nutrition through proper chewing.

3. Grooming and Toileting Supports

- **Nail clippers with extended handles**
- **Hairbrushes with ergonomic grips**
- **Incontinence pads, underwear, and mattress protectors**
- **Bidet toilet attachments** for increased hygiene and independence
- **Disposable hygiene wipes** (unscented and hypoallergenic)

Providing elders with the right tools can dramatically increase their confidence, comfort, and safety.

Hygiene and Elder Self-Esteem

Cleanliness is more than a physical condition—it's a psychological state that influences how we view ourselves. For the elderly, consistent hygiene is closely tied to **emotional well-being, personal dignity, and quality of life**.

1. The Psychological Benefits of Feeling Clean

- Boosts **confidence** in social situations (even within the family)
- Reduces **feelings of isolation or worthlessness**
- Encourages **better sleep and appetite**
- Supports **mood regulation**, especially in those with chronic illness or cognitive decline

Just as a child feels proud after learning to brush their own teeth, an elder feels more human when they are freshly washed, groomed, and dressed in clean clothes.

2. Hygiene as a Daily Anchor

In later life, routines are deeply comforting. Hygiene rituals, even when simplified, offer:

- **Structure in the day**
- **Purpose and participation**
- A way to stay **connected to the present moment**

Even if full bathing isn't possible daily, smaller acts—washing the face, brushing hair, applying lotion—can restore a sense of control and pride.

3. Encouraging Autonomy Where Possible

Elder hygiene care should not be "done to" the person—it should be **cooperative and respectful**. Encourage participation, even if minimal:

- "Would you like to choose the soap today?"
- "Can you wash your arms while I help with your back?"
- "Would you like to comb your own hair, or shall I help?"

The message should always be: **Your body is still yours. Your comfort still matters. You are still you.**

In Summary

Cleanliness in later years is not about appearance—it's about dignity, safety, comfort, and emotional resilience. The aging process presents undeniable challenges to personal hygiene, but with compassionate care, adaptive tools, and respectful support, these challenges can be met with grace and effectiveness.

When caregivers and loved ones prioritize hygiene in the elder years, they're not just helping someone bathe—they're helping them preserve their **identity, autonomy, and self-worth**.

Chapter 7: When We Neglect Cleanliness—The Real-Life Consequences

Cleanliness is often taken for granted until it's absent. When hygiene is neglected—whether temporarily due to stress or long-term due to physical, emotional, or cognitive challenges—the consequences ripple across every part of life. From physical health to social interaction, from emotional stability to long-term financial burdens, poor personal care has measurable and often painful impacts.

In this chapter, we dive into the tangible and intangible consequences of neglected hygiene. Far from a superficial matter, hygiene is a cornerstone of well-being, and its absence can silently erode a person's health, dignity, and place in the world.

Infections, Oral Disease, and Chronic Conditions

Hygiene is our first line of defense against illness. Neglecting it opens the door to preventable infections, skin disorders, dental decay, and exacerbation of existing chronic conditions.

1. Skin Infections

When the body isn't washed regularly, dirt, sweat, dead skin cells, and bacteria accumulate. This can result in:

- **Bacterial infections** like cellulitis or impetigo
- **Fungal infections** like athlete's foot, ringworm, and candidiasis
- **Dermatitis or eczema flare-ups** due to buildup of irritants and blocked pores
- **Infestations** of lice or scabies in severe cases

Minor skin issues, when untreated due to neglect, can become painful or even life-threatening in vulnerable populations.

2. Oral Health Problems

The mouth is home to hundreds of bacterial species, and without daily care, this microbial balance turns harmful. Poor oral hygiene leads to:

- **Tooth decay and cavities**
- **Gingivitis** (gum inflammation) progressing to **periodontitis**
- **Halitosis** (chronic bad breath)
- Increased risk of **oral infections**, tooth loss, and jawbone damage
- Evidence links **periodontal disease** to heart disease, stroke, and complications in diabetes

Teeth aren't just cosmetic—they are critical to nutrition, speech, and overall health.

3. Chronic Health Issues

Neglecting hygiene can worsen or trigger serious long-term health conditions, including:

- **Urinary tract infections** and kidney problems (especially in women and the elderly)
- **Respiratory infections** due to poor dental health or clogged nasal passages
- **Compounded complications** in diabetic patients with poor foot and skin care
- Higher rates of **hospital readmission** and longer recovery periods due to infections

In every stage of life, hygiene plays an essential role in **infection control, symptom management, and chronic disease prevention**.

The Mental Impact of Poor Hygiene

Poor hygiene doesn't just manifest on the body—it also deeply affects the mind. Whether it's a result of mental illness or a trigger for emotional distress, the relationship between hygiene and mental health is a powerful one.

1. Hygiene Neglect as a Symptom of Mental Illness

Many people struggling with mental health conditions report difficulty maintaining hygiene—not because they don't care, but because they're overwhelmed, fatigued, or emotionally shut down.

Common conditions associated with hygiene neglect include:

- **Major depressive disorder**
- **Post-traumatic stress disorder (PTSD)**
- **Schizophrenia and other psychotic disorders**
- **Anxiety disorders**
- **Bipolar disorder (especially during depressive episodes)**

In these cases, hygiene becomes an outward indicator of internal struggle.

2. Emotional Consequences of Feeling Unclean

Even without clinical depression, the act of being unclean can:

- Lower self-esteem
- Induce shame or self-disgust
- Increase avoidance behaviors (social withdrawal, staying indoors)
- Worsen body image issues
- Reinforce a negative self-perception

Cleanliness is closely tied to identity. A neglected appearance can make individuals feel invisible, devalued, or unworthy—leading to a vicious cycle of isolation and worsening self-care.

3. Hygiene and Cognitive Decline

For elderly individuals with dementia or cognitive impairment, hygiene routines may be forgotten, misunderstood, or resisted. Without compassionate support, hygiene decline can trigger confusion, fear, and further loss of independence.

Supporting hygiene for individuals with mental or cognitive disorders requires **sensitivity, structure, and nonjudgmental support**—not shame or punishment.

Social Rejection and Isolation

In a society that places high value on cleanliness, the consequences of visible hygiene neglect can be devastating to one's social life and relationships.

1. Stigma and Judgment

People who exhibit signs of poor hygiene may be:

- Teased, mocked, or bullied (especially children and teens)
- Avoided by peers, colleagues, or romantic partners
- Misunderstood as lazy or irresponsible
- Denied job opportunities, promotions, or fair treatment

The social penalty for poor hygiene is often disproportionate to the cause. Those struggling with hygiene due to poverty, disability, or mental illness are frequently met with **harsh judgment** rather than support.

2. Relationship Strain

Hygiene neglect can strain relationships in various ways:

- Intimate partners may feel uncomfortable, rejected, or disconnected
- Friends may distance themselves
- Family dynamics may become strained, especially when caregiving is involved

Poor hygiene becomes not just a personal issue—but a **relational and environmental burden** for those nearby.

3. Institutional Rejection

In more extreme cases, individuals with hygiene neglect may:

- Be **denied housing** in shelters or group homes
- Face **eviction or complaints** in shared housing
- Lose access to **employment or education** due to appearance or odor

This leads to systemic cycles of **homelessness, unemployment, and further marginalization**.

Long-Term Costs of Poor Personal Care

While hygiene may seem like a small detail in the scope of life, its neglect carries significant long-term consequences—both personally and societally.

1. Medical Costs

- Treating infections, oral disease, and preventable conditions costs **thousands of dollars annually**
- Hospitalization for skin ulcers, sepsis, or dental surgery due to neglect is **avoidable yet common**
- Lack of early hygiene intervention leads to **more expensive care needs** later

2. Dependency and Institutionalization

When personal hygiene declines, especially among the elderly or disabled, it often signals the need for:

- Assisted living or nursing care
- Professional home health aides
- Hospitalization or psychiatric evaluation

These are emotionally and financially taxing options that can be reduced with earlier hygiene support.

3. Intergenerational Effects

Children who grow up without hygiene guidance may internalize shame, suffer bullying, or carry poor habits into adulthood. In households where hygiene is neglected due to poverty or instability, children often bear long-term emotional and health scars.

Investment in hygiene education and support at every life stage can **prevent generational cycles of neglect**.

In Summary

When personal cleanliness is neglected, the consequences are not merely cosmetic—they are **medical, emotional, social, and economic**. Hygiene is not a luxury or vanity—it is a necessity tied to survival, self-worth, and public well-being.

By understanding the deep and wide-reaching impact of hygiene neglect, we can better advocate for early support, compassionate care, and systems that make cleanliness accessible to all—regardless of age, ability, or income.

Chapter 8: Hygiene and Mental Health—A Two-Way Street

Personal hygiene and mental health share a deeply reciprocal relationship. When one suffers, the other often follows. For many people, hygiene neglect isn't a conscious choice—it's a **symptom** of deeper emotional distress. Likewise, maintaining even the simplest hygiene routine can become a powerful anchor during times of psychological turmoil.

This chapter explores the dynamic between hygiene and mental health, shedding light on how emotional conditions affect self-care, and how re-establishing small rituals of cleanliness can support healing, dignity, and daily stability.

How Depression and Anxiety Affect Hygiene Habits

Mental health disorders like **depression, anxiety, PTSD, bipolar disorder, and schizophrenia** frequently impair a person's ability to maintain consistent hygiene. But the reasons are often misunderstood, misjudged, or minimized.

1. Depression and Hygiene Neglect

Depression is a condition of emotional exhaustion, cognitive fog, and often physical lethargy. What seems like a "simple shower" to a healthy person can feel like **climbing a mountain** to someone with depression.

Common barriers include:

- Lack of energy or motivation
- Feelings of hopelessness ("Why bother?")
- Executive dysfunction (difficulty initiating tasks)
- Shame or self-disgust that leads to avoidance
- Sensory sensitivity (e.g., water temperature, touch aversion)

For someone in a depressive episode, even brushing teeth can be overwhelming—not out of laziness, but out of survival-level fatigue.

2. Anxiety and Hygiene Distortion

While depression often results in hygiene neglect, anxiety can manifest in two extremes:

- **Avoidance-based neglect**, due to overstimulation, sensory discomfort, or paralysis in decision-making (e.g., overthinking which soap to use)
- **Compulsive hygiene**, where rituals like handwashing or grooming are repeated excessively as a form of control (common in OCD or health anxiety)

Anxiety-driven hygiene often stems from a **desire to feel safe**, but can spiral into stress when rituals become rigid or fear-based.

How Hygiene Routines Support Emotional Stability

While poor mental health can lead to neglected hygiene, the reverse is also true: **consistently practicing basic hygiene can improve mental health**. In this way, hygiene becomes a therapeutic tool.

1. Routine as a Grounding Mechanism

Daily hygiene tasks—brushing teeth, washing the face, combing hair—create **structure**, which is particularly important when life feels chaotic or overwhelming.

Benefits of a hygiene routine include:

- Providing **predictability** in uncertain times
- Reinforcing a sense of **accomplishment**
- Encouraging **executive functioning** through step-based tasks
- Marking transitions between emotional states (e.g., morning anxiety vs. post-shower calm)

These routines act like **emotional bookends**—starting and ending the day with care.

2. Cleanliness Boosts Mood and Self-Worth

Cleanliness often changes how we feel **about ourselves** and how we perceive the world around us. A warm shower, freshly brushed teeth, or clean clothes can shift mood instantly.

Emotional effects of hygiene include:

- **Elevated self-esteem**
- Greater **confidence in social settings**
- Sense of **pride and control**
- Reduction in physical discomfort or irritability

When we feel clean, we **reconnect with ourselves**—not as broken, but as cared for.

3. Hygiene as Emotional Regulation

Activities like bathing or moisturizing can activate the **parasympathetic nervous system**, calming the body's stress response. Warm water, soft textures, and repetitive movements all play a role in **lowering cortisol levels** and promoting a state of calm.

Mindful Grooming as Therapy

Hygiene doesn't need to be a clinical routine—it can become a **meditative and healing practice** when approached with mindfulness.

1. Sensory Awareness

Turn hygiene into a moment of **sensory grounding**:

- Notice the scent of shampoo
- Feel water running over your skin
- Listen to the sound of the toothbrush
- Observe how skin feels after applying lotion

These small acts shift your attention away from anxious thoughts and back into the **present moment**.

2. Self-Compassion in Action

Grooming is a physical way to **say "I care"** to your body. When done gently and without judgment, it becomes a mirror of emotional repair. Examples:

- Brushing hair as an act of tenderness
- Applying lotion to dry hands as a symbolic gesture of healing
- Washing the face as a ritual of renewal after crying or stress

These actions remind the mind: *You are not worthless. You are worthy of care.*

3. Reframing the Routine

Rather than viewing hygiene as a chore, reframe it as a **ceremony of care**:

- Use favorite products with pleasant textures or scents
- Set a calming playlist or podcast
- Light a candle or use soft lighting
- Pair hygiene time with positive affirmations ("I am taking care of myself today.")

Ritualizing these moments transforms them from duties into **restorative experiences**.

Supportive Hygiene Plans for Those Struggling Mentally

When mental health impairs hygiene, support plans should focus on **small wins, flexibility, and compassion**—not perfection.

1. Break It Down

Use **micro-goals** instead of complete routines:

- "Today, I'll wash my face and put on deodorant."
- "Tomorrow, I'll brush my teeth and change clothes."

Even doing one thing helps reestablish self-care momentum.

2. Use Visual and Verbal Cues

Create **hygiene checklists** or sticky notes in the bathroom. Use timers or phone reminders to:

- Brush teeth
- Take a shower
- Apply medication or skin treatments

Apps and smart home assistants can also offer gentle reminders.

3. Create a Hygiene Kit

Prepare a simple hygiene box or bag that contains:

- Toothbrush, toothpaste, floss
- Hairbrush, dry shampoo
- Face wipes or micellar water
- Travel-size lotion or deodorant
- Clean undergarments

Having everything in one place reduces decision fatigue and encourages spontaneous care.

4. Buddy Support and Gentle Accountability
Loved ones can assist with hygiene struggles **without shaming**. Try:

- "I'm going to shower—want to do it at the same time?"
- "Want me to bring you clean clothes?"
- "I made a hygiene checklist if you ever want help with routines."

Compassionate support reminds struggling individuals that **they are not alone** and that small acts still matter.

5. In-Home or Clinical Support
If hygiene neglect becomes severe, consider:

- Occupational therapy for adaptive hygiene tools
- In-home care for those with disabilities or mental health crises
- Outpatient mental health programs that integrate daily living routines

Addressing hygiene should always come **with empathy**, not discipline.

In Summary
Hygiene and mental health exist in a continuous, powerful feedback loop. Poor mental health can inhibit hygiene. Neglected hygiene can deepen emotional suffering. But small, intentional acts of grooming can serve as **bridges back to self-worth, presence, and recovery**.

We must begin to treat hygiene not merely as a physical task—but as a **mental health intervention**. Cleanliness is not about appearances. It's about honoring the self, even in the shadows.

Chapter 9: Hygiene in Public Health—Why It's Bigger Than Just You

Personal hygiene may seem like a private matter, but its impact extends far beyond the individual. Every hand washed, every sneeze contained, every clean surface maintained helps protect not only oneself but also the wider community. In fact, hygiene is one of the most powerful public health tools ever developed—simple, affordable, and highly effective.

This chapter explores how individual cleanliness contributes to community wellness, how infrastructure and policy uphold public hygiene standards, and why social responsibility is essential in maintaining safe, healthy environments.

Germ Spread, Pandemics, and Hygiene

In the face of communicable diseases, hygiene is a frontline defense. Viruses, bacteria, and fungi can spread quickly through air, surfaces, water, and skin contact—especially in crowded or shared environments.

1. How Germs Spread

Microorganisms are constantly transmitted through:

- **Touch** (e.g., shaking hands, shared objects)
- **Respiratory droplets** (from coughing, sneezing, or talking)
- **Surface contact** (e.g., doorknobs, handrails, elevator buttons)
- **Bodily fluids** (e.g., blood, saliva, or feces)

Pathogens that cause flu, colds, gastrointestinal illnesses, strep throat, and COVID-19 can survive on surfaces for hours or even days without hygiene intervention.

2. Lessons from Pandemics

Historically, hygiene has played a critical role in controlling and mitigating pandemics:

- During the **1918 flu pandemic**, handwashing and mask-wearing were emphasized alongside quarantine.
- The **cholera outbreaks** in the 19th century spurred the development of sewage systems and clean water access.
- The **COVID-19 pandemic** highlighted the importance of hand hygiene, surface disinfection, and respiratory etiquette.

Hygiene alone may not prevent disease outbreaks—but when combined with science-based policy and medical care, it **slows transmission**, reduces fatalities, and **saves lives**.

3. Key Public Health Hygiene Practices

- Handwashing with soap for at least 20 seconds
- Covering coughs and sneezes
- Cleaning frequently touched surfaces
- Staying home when sick
- Wearing masks when appropriate

These behaviors are **not just personal acts—they are public health contributions**.

Hygiene's Role in Public Infrastructure

Clean communities don't happen by accident—they're the result of **infrastructure, policy, and investment**. From water sanitation to waste management, public hygiene systems form the backbone of civilization.

1. Water Supply and Sanitation Systems

Clean water and sanitation access are essential human rights. Yet, billions still live without reliable plumbing or safe water sources.

Key infrastructure components:

- Municipal **water treatment plants**
- **Sewage systems** and septic tanks
- **Stormwater management**
- **Waste disposal and recycling** services

Breakdowns in these systems can lead to outbreaks of:

- Cholera
- Dysentery
- Hepatitis A
- Parasitic infections

Modern hygiene begins with **access**—to clean water, safe toilets, and efficient waste removal.

2. Urban Design and Cleanliness

Cities that prioritize public hygiene incorporate:

- Public restrooms and handwashing stations
- Trash and recycling bins in high-traffic areas
- Pest control and waste monitoring
- Air filtration in public buildings
- Green spaces that reduce pollution and improve respiratory health

Urban cleanliness **prevents disease and improves quality of life** for all citizens.

3. Funding and Regulation

Government health departments, environmental agencies, and urban planners all play roles in:

- Setting hygiene standards (e.g., water safety, restaurant inspections)
- Funding sanitation upgrades
- Responding to public health crises
- Enforcing cleanliness codes in housing and commercial buildings

Without policy and infrastructure, individual hygiene efforts are limited in effect. **Collective investment leads to collective health.**

Workplace and School Cleanliness Standards

Shared environments like offices, schools, and public transportation hubs are hotspots for illness transmission. Cleanliness in these spaces is not just a courtesy—it is a **legal and ethical responsibility**.

1. Workplace Hygiene

Employers have a duty to maintain a safe, clean, and health-conscious environment. Workplace hygiene includes:

- Regular cleaning and disinfecting of surfaces
- Stocking restrooms with soap, paper towels, and hand sanitizer
- Encouraging sick employees to stay home
- Promoting good hygiene practices through signage and training
- Providing clean air circulation and HVAC maintenance

In healthcare settings, hygiene is even more critical. Hospitals, clinics, and long-term care facilities must follow rigorous infection control protocols, including:

- Hand hygiene audits
- PPE usage
- Isolation procedures
- Sterile equipment handling

Poor workplace hygiene can result in absenteeism, legal liability, and reduced productivity.

2. School Hygiene

Children are particularly vulnerable to disease, and schools are prime sites for rapid germ spread.

Essential hygiene measures include:

- Teaching children to wash hands before meals and after restroom use
- Cleaning classrooms and shared equipment regularly
- Ensuring clean bathrooms and stocked supplies
- Encouraging students to stay home when sick
- Offering hygiene education in the curriculum

Schools that emphasize hygiene create healthier, happier learning environments and reduce sick days.

Social Responsibility and Community Hygiene

While systems and policies matter, hygiene is ultimately upheld by **individuals making mindful choices** that affect everyone around them.

1. Hygiene as Civic Duty

Practicing personal hygiene isn't just about you—it protects the elderly, the immunocompromised, young children, and people with chronic illnesses. These populations depend on the community to:

- Cover their mouths when coughing
- Wash hands after using public restrooms
- Dispose of waste properly
- Sanitize shared tools or equipment

Every hygienic action sends a message: *Your health matters to me.*

2. Reducing Stigma and Promoting Access

Cleanliness should not be a marker of wealth or privilege. Many people struggle with hygiene due to:

- Homelessness
- Physical or cognitive disabilities
- Financial limitations
- Lack of education or support

Community efforts can make hygiene accessible for all:

- Public showers and laundry facilities
- Free hygiene kits for unhoused individuals
- Educational programs in schools and community centers
- Compassion-based outreach, not judgment

Hygiene equality is a public health priority and a **moral imperative**.

3. Cultural and Global Collaboration

Hygiene standards and beliefs vary by culture. Global cooperation is vital in:

- Sharing best practices during pandemics
- Funding hygiene programs in underserved regions
- Respecting cultural hygiene rituals and adapting policies accordingly

Public hygiene is a **shared global responsibility**—from local towns to international cities.

In Summary

Clean hands can stop an epidemic. A well-stocked restroom can prevent an outbreak. A culture that values hygiene can uplift an entire generation.

Hygiene is not just personal—it is **collective, civic, and transformative**. Every community, workplace, school, and government has a role in promoting cleanliness and protecting health.

As we've seen, personal care has public consequences. The soap you use today could save someone's life tomorrow. It's not just about staying clean. It's about **caring for each other**.

Chapter 10: Sustainability and Hygiene—Clean Without Harm

As global awareness of environmental issues grows, so does the need to rethink how we stay clean. Hygiene, while essential to health and well-being, comes with a hidden environmental cost. From plastic packaging to water waste, many conventional hygiene practices leave a heavy footprint on the planet. But it doesn't have to be this way.

In this chapter, we examine the ecological impact of modern hygiene, explore eco-friendly alternatives, and offer practical steps for reducing your hygiene footprint—without compromising on cleanliness, comfort, or health. A truly clean body, after all, should not come at the expense of a polluted Earth.

Water Usage, Product Waste, and Environmental Cost

Maintaining hygiene consumes valuable natural resources, particularly water and materials used in product packaging. Over time, these daily habits contribute to climate stress, pollution, and overconsumption.

1. Water Waste in Hygiene Routines

Water is essential to personal cleanliness, but it's often used inefficiently.

Key statistics:

- A **10-minute shower** can use up to 25 gallons (95 liters) of water.
- Leaving the tap running while brushing your teeth can waste **up to 4 gallons per minute**.
- Bathing, shaving, and washing hair all contribute to **high daily water consumption**.

The cumulative impact is staggering, especially in regions where droughts and water scarcity are worsening.

2. Product Packaging and Plastic Pollution

Most hygiene products are packaged in **single-use plastic**:

- Shampoo and conditioner bottles
- Toothpaste tubes
- Deodorant containers
- Disposable razors and sanitary pads

Many of these items are **not recyclable** due to mixed materials or product residue. They end up in landfills or oceans, where they break down into **microplastics** that enter food chains, water supplies, and even human bloodstreams.

3. Toxic Ingredients and Environmental Runoff

Some personal care products contain **synthetic fragrances, microbeads, parabens, phthalates, and sulfates** that:

- Harm aquatic ecosystems
- Accumulate in wildlife
- Contaminate soil and water when washed down drains

The very act of washing ourselves can contribute to **polluting the planet**—unless we make smarter, more sustainable choices.

Green Alternatives: Shampoo Bars, Menstrual Cups, Bamboo Brushes

Fortunately, the eco-hygiene revolution is well underway. A growing number of individuals, brands, and movements are advocating for **clean hygiene that's clean for the Earth too**.

1. Solid and Low-Waste Products

- **Shampoo and conditioner bars** eliminate plastic bottles and last longer than liquid alternatives.
- **Bar soaps** packaged in paper or compostable wraps reduce plastic waste.
- **Toothpaste tablets** and **powders** offer plastic-free brushing options.
- **Reusable cotton rounds** or **face towels** replace disposable wipes and pads.

These products typically have a **lower carbon footprint**, use fewer resources, and generate less landfill waste.

2. Reusable Menstrual Products

- **Menstrual cups** are made of medical-grade silicone, last up to 10 years, and eliminate thousands of pads/tampons.
- **Reusable cloth pads** and **period underwear** offer sustainable alternatives to single-use products.
- These options also reduce exposure to bleach, plastic, and fragrance often found in disposable items.

Adopting these alternatives supports **menstrual equity** while dramatically reducing environmental harm.

3. Sustainable Grooming Tools

- **Bamboo toothbrushes** are biodegradable and compostable.
- **Safety razors** with replaceable blades eliminate plastic cartridges.
- **Wooden combs** and **natural bristle brushes** replace plastic grooming tools.
- **Metal tongue scrapers** and **glass floss containers** are long-lasting and eco-friendly.

These small swaps reduce plastic dependency while maintaining the same level of personal care.

4. Non-Toxic Ingredients and Clean Formulas

Eco-conscious consumers can seek out:

- **Fragrance-free** or naturally scented products
- Items labeled **biodegradable, organic,** or **cruelty-free**
- Brands that avoid **sodium lauryl sulfate, parabens, and microbeads**
- Refillable and bulk-buy options to reduce packaging

Buying better often means buying **less**, but more effectively.

How to Reduce Your Hygiene Footprint

Transitioning to sustainable hygiene is not about perfection—it's about **progress, awareness, and smarter choices**.

1. Audit Your Current Hygiene Habits

Start by asking:

- How much water do I use daily during hygiene tasks?
- Which products generate the most waste?
- What ingredients am I putting on my skin and into the environment?
- How often do I replace or discard hygiene tools?

Once aware, change becomes easier.

2. Simple Swaps for a Greener Routine

- Replace body wash with **bar soap**
- Switch to **reusable razors** or **safety razors**
- Turn off water while brushing teeth
- Use **biodegradable floss** and compostable cotton swabs
- Try **vinegar or baking soda-based cleaners** for surfaces and tools
- Buy **refillable bottles** or **bulk containers** where available

Each swap compounds over time, reducing landfill waste and conserving resources.

3. Extend the Life of What You Use

- Use only as much product as necessary—most people **overuse** shampoo, toothpaste, and cleanser.
- Clean and **store tools properly** to avoid mold or premature disposal.
- Repair or **refill containers** rather than throw them away.

Mindful usage is a quiet act of sustainability.

4. Support Green Brands and Local Makers

- Choose companies with **transparent sourcing and manufacturing practices**
- Support **small batch soap makers**, zero-waste stores, or farmers markets
- Avoid greenwashing by looking for **certifications** (e.g., B Corp, EWG Verified, Leaping Bunny)

Your dollar is a **vote for the future** you want to live in.

Clean Body, Clean Planet Philosophy

True hygiene isn't just about surface-level purity—it's about living in harmony with the world around us. As stewards of our health and the Earth's health, we must begin to view our hygiene rituals as **ecological acts** as much as personal ones.

1. Interconnected Wellness

- A clean planet supports human health—less pollution means fewer diseases.
- Natural skincare nourishes both **your body and the ecosystem** it returns to.
- Reducing consumption encourages **minimalism, gratitude, and clarity**.

Your hygiene routine becomes a daily **ritual of respect**—for yourself and for the Earth.

2. Teaching Sustainability Through Hygiene

Children and teens who grow up with sustainable hygiene learn:

- Personal responsibility
- Environmental awareness
- How to make ethical consumer choices

Every bar of soap, bamboo brush, or reusable product is an educational moment—a declaration that **cleanliness can be both personal and planetary**.

3. Collective Impact

If one person switches to a shampoo bar, it may not change the world. But if **millions do**, the plastic industry shifts. The landfills shrink. The oceans breathe easier.

Clean bodies shouldn't require a dirty planet. **It's time to clean without harm.**

In Summary

Sustainability and hygiene are not in conflict—they are part of the same goal: health. A clean planet is essential for clean living. And clean living, when done responsibly, helps protect the planet we call home.

By embracing eco-friendly habits, sustainable tools, and mindful consumption, you can reduce your environmental impact **one shower, one toothbrush, one product at a time**.

Chapter 11: Gender and Hygiene—Tailored Needs Across the Spectrum

Hygiene is a universal human need, but the way it manifests across genders is deeply influenced by biology, cultural norms, and social expectations. Men and women, as well as individuals across the gender spectrum, face distinct hygiene challenges—ranging from hormonal fluctuations and reproductive care to socially imposed grooming standards.

This chapter explores the **biological, emotional, and societal dimensions** of gender-specific hygiene. It emphasizes the importance of tailored care, the need to dismantle stereotypes, and the value of inclusive hygiene education that respects the needs of all bodies and identities.

Gender-Specific Challenges (Menstruation, Shaving, Facial Care)

Biological sex differences and gender roles influence personal care needs in key ways. While hygiene practices may overlap across genders, specific issues such as menstruation, hair grooming, and skincare routines often differ in both form and social meaning.

1. Menstruation Management (Primarily for Women and Some Non-Binary Individuals)

Menstrual hygiene is a central, recurring challenge for millions.
Key hygiene needs include:

- Regular changing of **sanitary products** (pads, tampons, menstrual cups, period underwear)
- **Handwashing before and after** handling menstrual products
- Cleaning of **reusable menstrual items** after each use
- Proper **disposal or sanitization** to prevent infections and odors

Challenges:

- Lack of access to menstrual hygiene products (often called "period poverty")
- Public shame or cultural taboos around menstruation
- Poor sanitation facilities in schools or workplaces

Solutions:

- Education around **safe menstrual practices**
- Promotion of **reusable, eco-friendly products**
- Inclusion of boys and men in menstrual awareness to reduce stigma

2. Shaving and Body Hair Maintenance

Shaving habits are strongly influenced by **gendered expectations**. These expectations are neither biologically mandated nor fixed.

- **Men** are typically expected to groom facial hair, and may shave or trim chest, back, or pubic hair.
- **Women** are often socially pressured to remove leg, underarm, facial, and bikini-area hair.

Hygiene concerns with shaving:

- Razor burn, ingrown hairs, skin infections
- Use of **clean, sharp blades**
- Application of **aftercare products** (moisturizer, antiseptic balms)

Cultural shift: More individuals are rejecting forced grooming norms and embracing **personal choice over social conformity**.

3. Facial and Skin Care Routines

Though everyone has skin, **gender-targeted marketing** often misrepresents skincare as a women-only concern.

- **Men's skin** is typically thicker, oilier, and more prone to irritation from shaving.
- **Women's skin** is more prone to hormonal acne and may change with menstrual cycles, pregnancy, or menopause.

Hygiene considerations:

- Use of **non-comedogenic**, gender-neutral products
- Encouraging all genders to moisturize, cleanse, and protect skin from UV exposure
- Destigmatizing skincare as **self-care for all humans**, not just beauty for women

Reproductive and Hormonal Hygiene Differences

Hormones and reproductive anatomy introduce distinct hygiene needs for individuals assigned male or female at birth.

1. Female Anatomy and Hormonal Changes

Women and people with female reproductive systems experience hormonal shifts across their lives—puberty, menstruation, pregnancy, postpartum, perimenopause, and menopause.

Key hygiene needs include:

- **External vulva cleaning** with water or gentle, pH-balanced products (avoid internal douching)
- Proper hygiene during menstruation, ovulation, and sexual activity
- Extra care during **pregnancy and postpartum** (e.g., perineal cleansing, breast care)
- Vaginal dryness and sensitivity during menopause may require **gentle moisturizers or lubricants**

Hygiene education must focus on **empowerment**, not shame or suppression.

2. Male Anatomy and Reproductive Hygiene

People with male reproductive anatomy also face unique needs. Hygiene considerations include:

- **Regular washing of the genital area**, including under the foreskin if uncircumcised
- Testicular hygiene and awareness of lumps, infections, or irritations
- Clean shaving of facial or body hair using proper tools
- Proper cleaning of any devices or aids used for erectile dysfunction or incontinence

Sexual and reproductive hygiene for men is often under-discussed, leading to misinformation and preventable health issues.

3. Hormonal Influence Across Genders

Hormonal fluctuations affect:

- **Sweat and odor production** (testosterone increases sweat gland activity)
- **Acne and skin oiliness**
- Mood, confidence, and motivation to engage in hygiene

For transgender individuals undergoing **hormone replacement therapy (HRT)**:

- Estrogen or testosterone therapy can lead to new skin, hair, and hygiene challenges
- Inclusive medical and hygiene guidance is essential to support trans individuals

Breaking Stereotypes in Men's and Women's Hygiene
Traditional gender roles have created rigid expectations for hygiene:

- Women are taught that **appearance equates to worth**
- Men are taught that **hygiene is feminine or optional**

These stereotypes harm everyone.

1. Harmful Messaging to Women

- Pressure to be hairless, poreless, and perpetually fresh
- Use of scented products that **disrupt vaginal pH**
- Shame around menstruation, body odor, or visible sweat
- Beauty disguised as hygiene—marketed grooming as necessity, not choice

This leads to **overconsumption, insecurity, and health risks** from over-cleansing or harsh products.

2. Harmful Messaging to Men

- Discouragement from skincare, grooming, or vulnerability
- Belief that "real men don't use lotion" or don't need to wash regularly
- Stigma around using hygiene products beyond soap and deodorant

This results in **neglect**, poor skin health, low confidence, and missed opportunities for self-care.

3. Moving Toward Balance

- Encourage **body autonomy**: each person chooses their own grooming path
- Promote **gender-neutral hygiene education** starting in early adolescence
- Value hygiene as a form of **health and respect**, not conformity

Everyone—regardless of gender—deserves to feel confident, comfortable, and informed about their body.

Inclusive Hygiene Education

To serve all people, hygiene education must be inclusive, respectful, and informed by diverse identities and experiences.

1. Teaching Beyond the Binary

Hygiene education should recognize:

- Non-binary and transgender individuals may have unique hygiene needs during transitions
- Not all women menstruate; not all men have facial hair
- All bodies, regardless of gender identity, require care and cleanliness

Curricula must include:

- Anatomy that reflects real-world diversity
- Safe, accurate information on **gender-affirming hygiene**
- Resources for **people with disabilities**, low-income individuals, and LGBTQ+ youth

2. Accessibility and Affirmation

Provide:

- Gender-neutral restrooms with free hygiene supplies
- Menstrual products in all bathrooms—not just women's
- Affirming signage that says "hygiene is for everyone"

Inclusive hygiene is **not political—it's human.**

3. Empowerment Over Enforcement

Rather than enforcing standards, encourage:

- Autonomy: "Here's what's healthy—you choose what works for you."
- Curiosity: "How does your body feel best cared for?"
- Empathy: "Everyone has different needs and experiences."

Inclusive hygiene education leads to **healthier, happier, and more respectful communities**.

In Summary

Gendered hygiene is about more than biology—it's about social messaging, bodily autonomy, and access to safe, affirming care. Whether managing menstruation, shaving, skincare, or hormonal shifts, people of all genders deserve **personalized support**, not pressure.

By breaking stereotypes, addressing diverse needs, and making hygiene inclusive, we foster a culture of self-respect, health, and empowerment for all.

Chapter 12: Culture and Cleanliness—Global Hygiene Practices

Cleanliness is a universal value, but the ways in which it is understood, practiced, and celebrated vary widely across cultures. Hygiene is not just a matter of biology—it is deeply rooted in **spirituality, history, geography, and social norms**. What one culture considers essential might be rare or even taboo in another. These differences do not reflect levels of "cleanliness," but rather the **diversity of human life and the cultural frameworks** that shape our habits.

This chapter explores global hygiene traditions—from daily rituals to sacred practices—revealing how people around the world maintain cleanliness and express respect for the body. It also emphasizes the importance of respecting cultural differences and how learning from these practices can deepen our understanding of hygiene as a rich, global heritage.

Cultural Hygiene Rituals Around the World

Cleanliness is often more than just a practical concern—it's spiritual, symbolic, and social. Across history, many cultures have developed hygiene routines that reflect beliefs about purity, honor, and identity.

1. Japan: Ritual Purity and Bathing

In Japan, hygiene is deeply embedded in both traditional and modern life.

- **Public baths (sento)** and **hot springs (onsen)** are popular for relaxation, community, and purification.
- Bathing is seen not just as cleaning the body, but as a ritual of **renewal and mental clarity**.
- One must always **wash and rinse thoroughly before entering shared water**, reflecting the cultural value of **not burdening others** with personal impurity.

Cleanliness is associated with order (*seiketsu*) and beauty (*kirei*), extending into daily life—from taking off shoes indoors to meticulous skincare and grooming.

2. India: Ayurveda, Oil Cleansing, and Spiritual Washing

In India, hygiene is closely tied to **Ayurveda**—a 5,000-year-old holistic health system.

- Daily routines include **oil pulling** (swishing oil in the mouth), **nasal cleansing (neti pots)**, and **tongue scraping**.
- **Abhyanga**, or full-body oil massage, is done regularly to promote circulation and detoxify the skin.
- Water plays a central role in purification; washing hands and feet before entering a home or temple is customary.
- Bathing before religious rituals or prayers is considered a **form of spiritual respect**.

Hygiene is seen as a balance of body, spirit, and energy.

3. Middle East: Ritual Washing (Wudu) in Islam

In Islamic tradition, **ritual cleanliness is foundational**.

- Muslims perform **wudu (ablution)** before prayer—washing the hands, face, arms, and feet with intention.
- **Ghusl**, a full-body wash, is required after specific spiritual or physical conditions.
- Cleanliness is closely linked with **spiritual readiness**, reflecting inner purity and submission to God.
- Using **water to cleanse after using the toilet** is a norm in many Islamic cultures—considered cleaner than toilet paper alone.

The emphasis on hygiene in Islam predates modern germ theory and is seen as both a **moral and practical command**.

4. Indigenous Cultures: Smoke, Steam, and Natural Elements

Many Indigenous traditions around the world include hygiene practices tied to **nature and healing**.

- **Sweat lodges** (in Native American and First Nations cultures) use heat and steam to cleanse body and spirit.
- **Smudging with herbs** like sage or cedar is believed to purify energy and surroundings.
- **Bark-based shampoos, clay masks, and herbal scrubs** are traditional skin and hair care techniques used in Africa, the Amazon, and Oceania.
- Hygiene is often viewed as **ritual maintenance** of harmony between humans and the environment.

These traditions emphasize **respect for the Earth** as the source of cleansing power.

Why Some Cultures Bathe Differently (or More Frequently)

Bathing frequency and method vary across cultures based on **climate, water access, cultural expectations, and historical beliefs.**

1. Climate and Water Access

- In **hot and humid regions**, people may bathe daily or even multiple times a day to stay cool and prevent skin infections.
- In **colder climates**, frequent bathing may be seen as unnecessary or even harmful due to dry skin or limited heating.
- In **rural or underdeveloped regions**, limited water infrastructure may reduce bathing frequency—but alternative methods like **wet cloth wiping, ash cleansing, or oil bathing** are used effectively.

2. Historical and Social Norms

- In parts of **Europe during the Middle Ages**, public bathing fell out of favor due to disease fears and moral codes. Dry hygiene (changing clothes, wiping the body) became common.
- In **modern Western societies**, daily showers are a norm—but often more cultural than medical. Dermatologists even warn against **over-bathing**, which can strip skin of protective oils.

Bathing frequency reflects **values, not superiority**. What matters is maintaining **health, comfort, and cultural integrity**.

3. Communal vs. Private Bathing

- Some cultures (like Turkey, Korea, Finland) embrace **communal bathing**, seeing it as bonding, therapeutic, and cleansing.
- Others emphasize **privacy**, associating nudity or body exposure with modesty or embarrassment.

Understanding these preferences helps promote **cultural sensitivity in shared spaces like gyms, spas, or refugee centers.**

Oral Hygiene, Foot Care, and Oiling Practices in Global Traditions

Many global hygiene customs target specific areas of the body and have been passed down through generations with scientific merit.

1. Oral Hygiene

- **Miswak (chewing sticks)** made from the Salvadora persica tree are widely used in the Middle East, Africa, and South Asia. They are naturally antibacterial and effective at cleaning teeth.
- In rural Latin America and Southeast Asia, **salt, charcoal, and coconut husk** are traditional tooth-cleaning agents.
- Ancient Mayans used **tree resin and herbs** for mouth cleansing.

Modern dental science now recognizes many of these practices as **beneficial and bio-compatible**.

2. Foot Washing and Footwear Traditions

- In many Asian, Middle Eastern, and African cultures, **shoes are removed before entering the home** to prevent bringing in dirt and spiritual impurity.
- **Foot washing** before prayer or sleep is common in Islamic, Indian, and Buddhist traditions.
- In some Native cultures, **barefoot grounding** is used to reconnect with the Earth's energy.

Feet are often **honored and cleansed**, reflecting humility, care, and sacred space.

3. Body Oiling and Skin Rituals

- In Africa and the Indian subcontinent, **shea butter, mustard oil, coconut oil, and neem oil** are used for skin nourishment and protection.
- Traditional Chinese medicine recommends **gua sha** (scraping the skin) and **moxibustion** to release toxins and increase circulation.
- Scandinavians practice **dry brushing** before saunas to exfoliate and stimulate lymphatic flow.

These practices are not just cosmetic—they serve as **preventative care and ritual renewal**.

Respecting and Learning from Other Norms

Understanding hygiene through a cultural lens opens the door to **mutual respect, empathy, and global awareness.**

1. Avoiding Ethnocentrism

- Judging another culture's hygiene by your own standards leads to misunderstanding and bias.
- Just because something is different doesn't mean it's inferior. **"Clean" is contextual.**

2. Cross-Cultural Learning

- Global hygiene wisdom is often **ahead of modern science.** Many ancient practices—like oil pulling, probiotic skincare, and natural deodorizers—are now gaining recognition in mainstream wellness.
- Openness to diverse practices encourages **hybrid solutions** that combine tradition with innovation.

3. Cultural Sensitivity in Global Communities

- In multicultural environments (schools, workplaces, hospitals), respect for diverse hygiene needs fosters inclusion.
- Offer **multiple options**: toilet paper and water, soap and oil, public and private spaces.
- Use **inclusive signage** and avoid shaming unfamiliar hygiene behaviors.

When we respect hygiene practices across cultures, we build **bridges, not barriers.**

In Summary

Hygiene is as diverse as humanity itself. Around the world, people stay clean through rituals shaped by **spiritual beliefs, climate, resources, and tradition**. Whether through steam baths, sacred oils, or communal practices, cleanliness reflects not just a body's health—but a culture's soul.

By learning from these traditions and respecting different norms, we broaden our understanding of hygiene as a **global human heritage**—one rooted in respect, dignity, and shared wellness.

Chapter 13: Technology and the Future of Hygiene

We are witnessing a revolution in hygiene—one driven not just by science, but by sensors, software, and smart devices. As technology becomes more deeply embedded in daily life, our personal hygiene habits are no longer static routines—they're evolving into **interactive, adaptive systems** that respond to our bodies in real-time.

This chapter explores the remarkable innovations shaping modern hygiene, from AI-driven skincare to wearables that monitor sweat composition. We'll also look ahead to the year 2050, forecasting how hygiene will be personalized, predictive, and even preventative in ways that seemed like science fiction only a few decades ago.

Smart Showers, Toothbrushes, and Skincare AI
Technology is transforming basic hygiene tools into intelligent allies.

1. Smart Showers
These next-generation bathing systems are engineered for comfort, efficiency, and data feedback:

- **Customizable profiles** for individuals: temperature, pressure, and duration presets.
- **Water conservation algorithms** track your usage and reduce waste automatically.
- **LED indicators** guide you through a time-optimized shower for energy and skin health.
- Some models integrate **aromatherapy or UV sanitation features** for full-body renewal.

These devices don't just clean the body—they help build smarter habits, monitor hygiene consistency, and support environmental goals.

2. Smart Toothbrushes
Toothbrushing has become data-rich with innovations like:

- **Built-in pressure sensors** that alert users if they brush too hard (which can damage gums).
- **Bluetooth connectivity** that syncs to apps, offering visual maps of missed spots.
- **AI coaching** that provides personalized tips based on brushing patterns.
- Some models now link with **dentist dashboards**, offering remote hygiene assessments.

This gamification of brushing boosts oral hygiene while giving real-time feedback—especially useful for children or the elderly.

3. Skincare AI and Facial Mapping

AI-based skincare apps and devices use facial scans to:

- **Assess pores, hydration, oil levels, redness, and fine lines** in seconds.
- Recommend personalized product routines based on real-time skin conditions.
- Track progress over days or weeks, improving consistency and early detection of skin issues.
- Advanced devices even dispense custom moisturizers or serums **based on daily scans.**

AI doesn't just enhance skincare—it **empowers self-awareness** and long-term skin health management.

Innovations in Deodorants, Wearables, and Trackers

Beyond cleaning, modern hygiene is about **monitoring, prevention, and adaptation**.

1. Next-Gen Deodorants

Today's deodorants are more than scent-masking sticks:

- **pH-sensitive formulas** adapt to body chemistry for longer-lasting protection.
- **Microbiome-friendly products** preserve good skin bacteria while neutralizing odor.
- **Smart deodorant dispensers** sync with apps and offer refill reminders, usage stats, and product recommendations.
- Some brands now offer **DNA-based customization**—analyzing your unique odor profile to create a personalized blend.

These innovations address hygiene at a molecular level.

2. Hygiene-Tracking Wearables

New wearables don't just count steps—they evaluate cleanliness:

- **Sweat sensors** detect dehydration, electrolyte imbalances, and signs of illness.
- Devices worn on the skin or in clothing can monitor **temperature, pH, moisture, and bacterial growth**.
- Hygiene alerts can warn about **excessive sweat, missed handwashing**, or the need to reapply skincare.
- Future clothing may integrate **antibacterial fibers** and **self-cleaning fabrics** using nanotechnology.

These tools provide **real-time feedback on hygiene-related health metrics**, closing the gap between routine and medical care.

3. Air and Surface Hygiene Monitors

Environmental hygiene is also evolving:

- **Air purifiers with pathogen sensors** detect bacteria, allergens, and VOCs (volatile organic compounds).
- **Touch-surface trackers** in public or shared spaces assess cleanliness based on microbial load.
- These innovations help **ensure hygiene beyond the body**—especially critical in hospitals, schools, and homes with immuno-compromised individuals.

The future of hygiene extends beyond self—it becomes **environmentally responsive**.

Hygiene as Biofeedback for Health

Hygiene is becoming more than a habit—it's a **diagnostic tool**.

1. Early Detection Through Hygiene Data

- Unusual body odor or sweat composition can signal **diabetes, infections, or hormonal imbalances.**
- Changes in dental hygiene patterns or gum color can point to **systemic inflammation** or heart conditions.
- Skin sensors may detect **UV damage, vitamin deficiencies, or dehydration** before symptoms appear.

Personal hygiene products and devices now serve as **first-line health surveillance systems.**

2. Mental Health Insights from Hygiene Patterns

- AI-driven hygiene apps can **track changes in grooming behavior**, helping identify depressive episodes early.
- Missed showers, skipped brushing, or reduced self-care may signal **emotional or cognitive decline.**
- Connected devices can notify caregivers or therapists—enabling **compassionate intervention without surveillance.**

In this sense, hygiene becomes a **mirror to emotional well-being** as much as physical health.

What Hygiene Will Look Like in 2050

By 2050, hygiene will be **frictionless, predictive, and integrated** into every aspect of life.

1. Personalized Hygiene Capsules

- Morning hygiene may occur in a **fully automated pod** that scans your body, applies personalized cleansing mists, oils, UV light treatments, and air-drying—no soap or towels required.
- Products will be tailored based on **your DNA, environment, and real-time health data**.

2. AI-Guided Hygiene Coaches

- Digital assistants will monitor your daily hygiene, recommend adjustments, and **order supplies automatically** based on behavior and biometrics.
- They will adapt based on **climate, stress levels, activity, and social calendar** (e.g., deeper cleanse before a big event).

3. Nanotech and Molecular Hygiene

- **Self-cleaning skin sprays** may protect the microbiome while repelling pathogens.
- **Internal health monitors** will inform external hygiene (e.g., warning you to hydrate, moisturize, or wash based on your sweat's chemical composition).
- **Nanobots** could one day clean teeth, pores, and wounds at the cellular level.

4. Environmentally Integrated Hygiene

- Smart homes will remind you to wash hands when returning home, clean your air, and sanitize shared items.
- **Public transport, gyms, and workplaces** will use passive hygiene systems—UV-cleaning seats, antimicrobial handrails, and touchless sterilization zones.

Cleanliness will become **automatic, adaptive, and intuitive**.

In Summary

Technology is transforming hygiene from routine maintenance into a **personalized wellness system**. Smart devices, AI coaches, and biofeedback tools are making it possible to understand, refine, and enhance cleanliness like never before.

In the future, hygiene will not just be about being clean—it will be about being **in sync** with your biology, your surroundings, and your emotional health. As we integrate data, automation, and customization into our hygiene habits, we move closer to a world where cleanliness is not just a private act, but a **public, digital, and deeply human evolution.**

Chapter 14: Teaching Cleanliness—Parenting, Caregiving, and Role Modeling

Cleanliness is not merely a task—it is a life skill. Teaching it, however, is not just about conveying rules and routines; it's about **modeling, guiding, and empowering** others to care for their bodies with dignity and autonomy. Whether you're a parent, caregiver, teacher, or support worker, your approach to hygiene education can shape someone's relationship with their body for a lifetime.

This chapter explores the art of teaching hygiene at every stage of life, with a special emphasis on **compassionate communication, adaptive methods, and the emotional side of self-care**. We dive into best practices for role modeling hygiene for children, supporting it in vulnerable populations, and fostering environments where hygiene education is not about shame, but about self-respect and love.

How to Model Hygiene for Children and Teens

Children learn hygiene not just by being told what to do—but by watching what those around them *do consistently*. Role modeling is one of the most powerful educational tools.

1. Be a Living Example

- **Consistency matters**: Children mimic what they see. When adults bathe regularly, brush their teeth, wash hands after using the restroom, or wear deodorant, children internalize these as standard habits.
- Use **visible routines**: Let children see you brushing, flossing, washing your face, and clipping your nails. Even folding clean clothes reinforces hygiene as part of life.
- Narrate your actions in age-appropriate ways: "I'm brushing my teeth to keep my smile healthy," or "I'm putting on deodorant so I don't smell bad later today."

2. Integrate Hygiene into Family Rituals

- **Make hygiene interactive**: Set a timer for brushing, sing songs during handwashing, and turn bath time into play.
- Reinforce through **positive feedback**: "Your hair smells so clean!" or "You did a great job washing your hands after playing outside."
- Use **visual charts** with stickers or tokens for kids who thrive on structure and rewards.

3. Talk About Puberty Before It Happens

For preteens and teens, hygiene can become awkward—but proactive conversations build confidence:

- Normalize body changes (sweating, acne, menstruation) before they happen.
- Offer **gender-affirming hygiene kits** with deodorant, razors, pads, skincare, etc.
- Emphasize hygiene as self-respect, not just a way to "avoid being gross."

Avoid criticizing appearance. Instead, teach that hygiene is a way to *feel good and in control* of their changing body.

Supporting Hygiene in Disabled or Elderly Relatives

Cleanliness is a right—not a privilege reserved for the young and able-bodied. For those who live with physical, cognitive, or emotional limitations, **maintaining hygiene may require support, compassion, and creative solutions**.

1. Understand the Individual's Capabilities

- Some may need **full assistance**, while others benefit from tools that increase independence (e.g., long-handled sponges, no-rinse shampoo caps, adaptive toothbrushes).
- Involve the person in decision-making where possible: "Would you like help today, or would you prefer to try on your own first?"
- Respect their dignity. Avoid infantilizing tone or excessive control.

2. Adapt the Environment

- Install **grab bars, shower chairs, non-slip mats**, and other safety equipment to create confidence in hygiene spaces.
- Use **visual guides or checklists** for individuals with memory challenges.
- Keep supplies visible, reachable, and simplified (color-coded bins, pump bottles instead of screw-tops).

3. Create a Compassionate Routine

- Predictability reduces stress. Establish **daily or weekly hygiene schedules**.
- Offer **choices whenever possible** to foster autonomy: "Do you want to bathe before or after breakfast?"
- Use **music, aromatherapy, or calming conversation** during hygiene tasks to make the experience enjoyable and familiar.

Remember: The goal isn't perfection—it's preserving **comfort, cleanliness, and self-worth**.

Remember: The goal isn't perfection—it's preserving **comfort, cleanliness, and self-worth**.

Empowering Instead of Shaming

Too often, hygiene education is linked with embarrassment or judgment. This damages self-esteem and can lead to **avoidance, secrecy, or defiance**.

1. Words Matter

Avoid:

- "You stink."
- "You look disgusting."
- "Why are you so dirty?"

Try instead:

- "Let's freshen up—you'll feel better."
- "I noticed your hair is oily—want help washing it tonight?"
- "Do you want to talk about ways to manage your skin?"

Use language that **uplifts, guides, and reassures**.

2. Don't Make Cleanliness a Moral Issue

Cleanliness is a *health habit*, not a reflection of personal virtue. Avoid equating dirtiness with laziness, worthlessness, or sin.

- Life gets messy—especially in poverty, disability, or depression.
- Offer **compassion and support**, not guilt or ultimatums.
- Praise effort over outcome: "I'm proud you brushed today, even if it was hard."

3. Build Intrinsic Motivation

Teach hygiene as a way to:

- Feel refreshed
- Prevent illness
- Show self-care
- Respect shared spaces

Let individuals **own their hygiene habits**, instead of doing them solely to avoid punishment or peer rejection.

Teaching Hygiene Compassionately in Schools

Schools are a powerful setting to reinforce hygiene—but how it's taught matters greatly.

1. Go Beyond "Wash Your Hands"

Many hygiene lessons stop at basic slogans. Instead, provide:

- Age-appropriate **discussions about puberty, oral care, skincare, and body odor**
- **Interactive learning tools** (posters, videos, hygiene stations, kits)
- **Inclusive messaging** that acknowledges different cultural, gender, and disability needs

2. Normalize, Don't Stigmatize

- Avoid using peer shaming (e.g., "Nobody wants to be around someone who smells").
- Encourage open, safe conversations about hygiene questions and challenges.
- Offer **private access to supplies** (deodorant, menstrual pads, toothpaste) without making students ask.

3. Involve Families and Caregivers

Send home hygiene information and resources that respect diverse backgrounds.

- Partner with local clinics or programs to offer **free hygiene kits**.
- Translate materials and **avoid one-size-fits-all messaging**.

By building a **community of support around hygiene**, schools become safer, more compassionate spaces for growing up.

In Summary

Teaching cleanliness is about **guidance, not enforcement**. Whether you're nurturing toddlers, supporting elders, or mentoring teens, your approach to hygiene education has lifelong impact.

When we model healthy habits, adapt support for unique needs, and replace shame with empowerment, we help others form a **resilient and respectful relationship with their bodies**. Cleanliness then becomes more than just soap and water—it becomes an expression of dignity, care, and compassion across generations.

Chapter 15: Clean Body, Clear Mind, Confident Life

Cleanliness is not just about physical wellness. It's a force that radiates through your confidence, mood, energy levels, and the way you face the world. When you feel clean, you move differently. You speak with more assurance. You meet the day with clarity rather than chaos. Cleanliness is foundational to how you live—and how you lead.

This final chapter explores the deep link between hygiene and self-esteem, posture, focus, and even **energetic or spiritual alignment**. We'll also share simple but powerful daily rituals that transform hygiene into an act of empowerment. Whether you're beginning your self-care journey or looking to build a hygiene legacy for future generations, this is where it all comes together.

How Hygiene Affects Posture, Confidence, and Productivity

Hygiene may start in the bathroom—but its impact is visible in every area of your life.

1. Posture and Body Language

Feeling clean alters how you carry yourself:

- Clean skin and fresh clothing can subconsciously promote **open posture**, lifted shoulders, and a relaxed stance.
- People who are unshowered or in stained clothes tend to **hunch, avoid eye contact**, or shrink into themselves.
- Cleanliness promotes **presence**—a feeling that you belong in the room, not that you're trying to hide.

Even a simple shower or fresh set of clothes can instantly **reset your physical confidence.**

2. Confidence and Self-Worth

- Cleanliness reinforces the belief: **"I'm worth taking care of."**
- When you regularly invest time in your hygiene, your brain interprets this as self-respect.
- The reverse is also true—neglecting hygiene can lead to a **reinforcement of low self-worth** or internalized shame.

By cleaning your body, you are reminding yourself: **"I deserve care."**

3. Hygiene and Daily Productivity

- Cleanliness rituals create **structure**. A morning shower or evening grooming ritual creates rhythm and intention.
- Many high performers report that **a clean start leads to clearer focus**, faster task execution, and fewer distractions.
- Smelling fresh, brushing your teeth, and having clean hands primes your body to be more **awake and responsive**—ready to engage rather than retreat.

Cleanliness is a subtle yet powerful catalyst for action.

Cleanliness and Spiritual or Energetic Wellbeing

In nearly every culture and spiritual path, cleanliness has long been considered a form of **inner purification**.

1. Energy and Aura

- Many believe that regular bathing or washing dispels **stagnant energy** or emotional residue from stressful environments.
- Practices like **salt baths, essential oil showers, or brushing off energy** are used to restore vitality and balance.
- Energetically, being clean is associated with **openness, receptivity, and protection**.

Even for those outside spiritual traditions, a clean body often translates to a **lightened emotional state**—a kind of psychological detox.

2. Ritual and Reverence

- Morning hygiene can be done with mindfulness and intention: "I wash away yesterday's fear and prepare to lead with clarity."
- Evening rituals can signal closure: "As I clean my body, I release this day and return to peace."
- Touching your own skin with intention—when brushing, washing, or moisturizing—can become a **meditative form of self-connection**.

These rituals reinforce the idea that hygiene is more than maintenance. It's **sacred attention**.

Morning/Evening Hygiene Rituals for Life Transformation

The way you start and end your day can change your mindset, relationships, and energy levels over time. Ritualizing hygiene gives structure and meaning to your daily rhythm.

Morning Ritual (Energize and Empower)

1. **Hydrate**: Drink water with lemon or minerals before any caffeine or food.
2. **Dry Brush or Stretch**: Stimulate your lymph system and awaken your circulation.
3. **Shower with Intention**: Use invigorating scents (e.g., citrus, mint), and visualize cleansing stress or lethargy.
4. **Skin + Oral Routine**: Gentle facial cleanse, moisturize, floss, and brush.
5. **Dress to Respect**: Even on off days, wear clothes that reflect care and readiness.

These 5 steps take 20–30 minutes and **set a tone of self-respect and clarity** for the entire day.

Evening Ritual (Release and Rebuild)

1. **Unwind with Warm Water**: A bath, a hot towel rubdown, or even a foot soak.
2. **Oil or Moisturize the Skin**: Especially hands, face, and feet—restore and soothe.
3. **Oral Care with Gratitude**: Brushing and flossing as a thank-you to the body that served you all day.
4. **Clean Environment**: Tidy your space briefly—external hygiene mirrors inner clarity.
5. **Mindful Closure**: End the day with a deep breath, prayer, or intention for healing rest.

These habits reprogram your brain and body for **deep rest, regeneration, and inner peace**.

Final Tips for Building a Lifelong Hygiene Legacy

Leaving behind a hygiene legacy doesn't mean being perfect. It means living in a way that honors the body and teaches others how to do the same.

1. Simplify and Personalize

- Your hygiene routine should feel achievable, not overwhelming.
- Find products and rituals that reflect your skin, culture, budget, and schedule.
- Don't compare your self-care to others—**consistency beats complexity**.

2. Stay Flexible Through Life Changes

- Life phases—pregnancy, disability, depression, elderhood—will affect hygiene.
- Adapt tools and timelines instead of abandoning routines altogether.
- Remember: Even a 5-minute wash or face splash is an act of self-respect.

3. Pass It On

- Model hygiene for your kids, partner, students, or those you care for.
- Make it **visible, positive, and emotionally safe**.
- Share rituals that uplift, not control.

4. Let Hygiene Be Healing

- When life feels chaotic, start with washing your hands.
- When you feel disconnected, brush your hair slowly.
- When you're overwhelmed, shower away the noise.

You don't need to wait to "fix your life" before caring for your body. Often, it begins **the other way around**.

In Summary

Cleanliness is more than skin-deep—it is the foundation of confidence, clarity, and self-respect. Whether it's preparing you for a job interview, calming your nervous system before bed, or giving you a reason to get out of bed on a hard day—hygiene is your daily reset button.

With a clean body comes a clear mind.
With a clear mind comes a confident life.

May your hygiene journey be more than just habit. May it be a form of **personal power, peaceful ritual, and generational legacy.**

Appendix A: Hygiene Essentials by Age Group

Cleanliness is not one-size-fits-all. Each stage of life presents unique physical, emotional, and practical hygiene needs. The products and tools that support good hygiene must be tailored to a person's developmental abilities, body changes, living environment, and sense of dignity.

This appendix outlines the most essential hygiene items across four key life stages—infancy and childhood, adolescence, adulthood, and elderhood. These curated recommendations include both **basic necessities and thoughtful extras** to promote independence, comfort, and confidence at every age.

Infants and Children (Ages 0–12)

In these early years, hygiene is about **gentle care, fun engagement, and forming positive routines**. Products should prioritize safety, comfort, and playful encouragement to make cleanliness enjoyable rather than stressful.

Essentials:

- **Tear-Free Shampoo & Mild Soap:**
  Formulas made for sensitive skin and eyes reduce bath time resistance and minimize irritation.
- **Soft Hair and Body Brushes:**
  Ideal for cradle cap or gentle exfoliation; use silicone or extra-soft bristles.
- **Colorful Toothbrushes & Flossers:**
  Featuring favorite characters, lights, or timers to encourage brushing habits.
- **Training Potty Hygiene:**
  Flushable wipes, step stools, and toilet training seats help ease the transition with minimal mess.
- **Wet Wipes & Diapering Supplies:**
  Hypoallergenic wipes, diaper creams, and antibacterial hand gel for caregivers.
- **Fun Towels & Bath Toys:**
  Hooded towels, themed washcloths, and squirting toys make bath time feel like playtime.

Pro Tip: Use a reward chart to reinforce hygiene tasks like brushing teeth, washing hands, or learning to bathe independently.

Teens (Ages 13–19)

Puberty brings rapid physical and emotional changes. Hygiene tools for teens should support **acne management, body odor control, and the growing need for privacy and autonomy**.

Essentials:

- **Acne Care Kits:**
  Include face washes with salicylic acid or benzoyl peroxide, gentle exfoliants, and pimple patches.
- **Deodorant (Natural & Antiperspirant Options):**
  Offer a choice to explore what feels comfortable—gel, stick, or spray.
- **Menstrual Hygiene Products:**
  Pads, tampons, menstrual cups, heating pads, and discreet carry cases for school days.
- **Shaving Kits:**
  Razors (manual or electric), shaving cream, aftercare products, and tips for safe shaving.
- **Electric Toothbrushes with Timers:**
  Help teens maintain consistency while improving dental health.
- **Face Cleansers & Moisturizers:**
  Products geared toward oily or combination skin types, free from heavy fragrances.
- **Self-Care Planners or Skincare Calendars:**
  Visual reminders for skincare routines, oral care, and menstrual tracking.

Pro Tip: Respect privacy and normalize open conversations about bodily changes to empower hygiene confidence.

Adults (Ages 20–59)

Adulthood hygiene is about **efficiency, customization, and stress relief.** Products should support busy schedules while encouraging deeper self-care and adaptability for different roles—worker, parent, traveler, or caregiver.

Essentials:

- **Complete Grooming Kits:**
  Nail clippers, tweezers, razors, trimmers, and mirrors for on-the-go or home use.
- **Dental Hygiene Sets:**
  Electric or ultrasonic toothbrushes, floss picks, tongue scrapers, and whitening kits.
- **Personalized Skincare Regimens:**
  Anti-aging serums, SPF moisturizers, exfoliators, and cleansers based on skin type or concerns.
- **Reusable Hygiene Products:**
  Travel toiletry kits, menstrual cups, silicone ear swabs, refillable containers.
- **Stress-Relieving Accessories:**
  Aromatherapy diffusers, Epsom salts, bath bombs, shower steamers, or eye masks.
- **Eco-Friendly Upgrades:**
  Bamboo toothbrushes, zero-waste soap bars, sustainable packaging.

Pro Tip: Pair hygiene habits with mindfulness (e.g., deep breathing in the shower) to turn routine into daily restoration.

Elderly (Ages 60+)

Later-life hygiene must address **mobility limitations, sensitive skin, safety concerns, and dignity preservation**. Comfort, accessibility, and emotional support are essential.

Essentials:

- **No-Slip Shower Mats & Grab Bars:**
  Help prevent falls and increase confidence in bathing independently.
- **Sponge Bathing Tools & Rinse-Free Cleansers:**
  Allow for waterless cleansing on days when showering is not feasible.
- **Moisturizing Soaps & Hypoallergenic Lotions:**
  Protect thin, delicate skin from drying or cracking.
- **Easy-Grip Nail Tools & Magnifying Mirrors:**
  Help maintain grooming when fine motor skills decline.
- **Long-Handled Brushes & Toe-Washing Aids:**
  Reduce bending or straining during bathing routines.
- **Soft Bristle Toothbrushes & Denture Care Supplies:**
  Include denture baths, brushes, and gentle toothpaste formulas.

Pro Tip: Hygiene routines can be emotionally sensitive—always prioritize **dignity, privacy, and patient pacing** during care.

In Summary

Having the right hygiene tools for each life stage isn't just about convenience—it's about **empowering self-care, preserving independence, and enhancing confidence**. By investing in age-appropriate essentials, we don't just support physical cleanliness—we affirm the value of each individual, no matter their age or ability.

As you continue your personal hygiene journey or guide others through theirs, let this appendix be a reminder: **the tools we choose shape the habits we form—and those habits shape the lives we lead.**

<u>Message from the Author:</u>

I hope you enjoyed this book, I love astrology and knew there was not a book such as this out on the shelf. I love metaphysical items as well. Please check out my other books:

-Life of Government Benefits

-My life of Hell

-My life with Hydrocephalus

-Red Sky

-World Domination:Woman's rule

-World Domination:Woman's Rule 2: The War

-Life and Banishment of Apophis: book 1

-The Kidney Friendly Diet

-The Ultimate Hemp Cookbook

-Creating a Dispensary(legally)

-Cleanliness throughout life: the importance of showering from childhood to adulthood.

-Strong Roots: The Risks of Overcoddling children

-Hemp Horoscopes: Cosmic Insights and Earthly Healing

- Celestial Hemp Navigating the Zodiac: Through the Green Cosmos

-Astrological Hemp: Aligning The Stars with Earth's Ancient Herb

-The Astrological Guide to Hemp: Stars, Signs, and Sacred Leaves

-Green Growth: Innovative Marketing Strategies for your Hemp Products and Dispensary

-Cosmic Cannabis

-Astrological Munchies

-Henry The Hemp

-Zodiacal Roots: The Astrological Soul Of Hemp

- **Green Constellations: Intersection of Hemp and Zodiac**

-Hemp in The Houses: An astrological Adventure Through The Cannabis Galaxy

-Galactic Ganja Guide

Heavenly Hemp

Zodiac Leaves

Doctor Who Astrology

Cannastrology

Stellar Satvias and Cosmic Indicas

Celestial Cannabis: A Zodiac Journey

AstroHerbology: The Sky and The Soil: Volume 1

AstroHerbology:Celestial Cannabis:Volume 2

Cosmic Cannabis Cultivation

The Starry Guide to Herbal Harmony: Volume 1

The Starry Guide to Herbal Harmony: Cannabis Universe: Volume 2

Yugioh Astrology: Astrological Guide to Deck, Duels and more

Nightmare Mansion: Echoes of The Abyss

Nightmare Mansion 2: Legacy of Shadows

Nightmare Mansion 3: Shadows of the Forgotten

Nightmare Mansion 4: Echoes of the Damned

The Life and Banishment of Apophis: Book 2

Nightmare Mansion: Halls of Despair

Healing with Herb: Cannabis and Hydrocephalus

Planetary Pot: Aligning with Astrological Herbs: Volume 1

Fast Track to Freedom: 30 Days to Financial Independence Using AI, Assets, and Agile Hustles

Cosmic Hemp Pathways

How to Become Financially Free in 30 Days: 10,000 Paths to Prosperity

Zodiacal Herbage: Astrological Insights: Volume 1

Nightmare Mansion: Whispers in the Walls

The Daleks Invade Atlantis

Henry the hemp and Hydrocephalus

10X The Kidney Friendly Diet

Cannabis Universe: Adult coloring book

Hemp Astrology: The Healing Power of the Stars

Zodiacal Herbage: Astrological Insights: Cannabis Universe: Volume 2

<u>Planetary Pot: Aligning with Astrological Herbs: Cannabis Universes: Volume 2</u>

Doctor Who Meets the Replicators and SG-1: The Ultimate Battle for Survival

Nightmare Mansion: Curse of the Blood Moon

<u>The Celestial Stoner: A Guide to the Zodiac</u>

Cosmic Pleasures: Sex Toy Astrology for Every Sign

Hydrocephalus Astrology: Navigating the Stars and Healing Waters

Lapis and the Mischievous Chocolate Bar

Celestial Positions: Sexual Astrology for Every Sign

Apophis's Shadow Work Journal: **:** A Journey of Self-Discovery and Healing

Kinky Cosmos: Sexual Kink Astrology for Every Sign

Digital Cosmos: The Astrological Digimon Compendium

Stellar Seeds: The Cosmic Guide to Growing with Astrology

Apophis's Daily Gratitude Journal

Cat Astrology: Feline Mysteries of the Cosmos

The Cosmic Kama Sutra: An Astrological Guide to Sexual Positions

Unleash Your Potential: A Guided Journal Powered by AI Insights

Whispers of the Enchanted Grove

Cosmic Pleasures: An Astrological Guide to Sexual Kinks

369, 12 Manifestation Journal

Whisper of the nocturne journal(blank journal for writing or drawing)

The Boogey Book

Locked In Reflection: A Chastity Journey Through Locktober

Generating Wealth Quickly:How to Generate $100,000 in 24 Hours

Star Magic: Harness the Power of the Universe

The Flatulence Chronicles: A Fart Journal for Self-Discovery

The Doctor and The Death Moth

Seize the Day: A Personal Seizure Tracking Journal

The Ultimate Boogeyman Safari: A Journey into the Boogie World and Beyond

Whispers of Samhain: 1,000 Spells of Love, Luck, and Lunar Magic: Samhain Spell Book

Apophis's guides:Witch's Spellbook Crafting Guide for Halloween

<u>Frost & Flame: The Enchanted Yule Grimoire of 1000 Winter Spells</u>

<u>The Ultimate Boogey Goo Guide & Spooky Activities for Halloween Fun</u>

Harmony of the Scales: A Libra's Spellcraft for Balance and Beauty

The Enchanted Advent: 36 Days of Christmas Wonders

Nightmare Mansion: The Labyrinth of Screams

Harvest of Enchantment: 1,000 Spells of Gratitude, Love, and Fortune for Thanksgiving

The Boogey Chronicles: A Journal of Nightly Encounters and Shadowy Secrets

The 12 Days of Financial Freedom: A Step-by-Step Christmas Countdown to Transform Your Finances

Sigil of the Eternal Spiral Blank Journal

A Christmas Feast: Timeless Recipes for Every Meal

Holiday Stress-Free Solutions: A Survival Guide to Thriving During the Festive Season

Whispers of the Harvest: The Corn Mother's Journal

The Evergreen Spellbook

The Doctor Meets the Boogeyman

The White Witch of Rose Hall's SpellBook

The Gingerbread Golem's Shadow: A Study in Sweet Darkness

The Gingerbread Golem Codex: An Academic Exploration of Sweet Myths

The Gingerbread Golem Grimoire: Sweet Magicks and Spells for the Festive Witch

The Curse of the Gingerbread Golem

10-minute Christmas Crafts for kids

<u>Christmas Crisis Solutions: The Ultimate Last-Minute Survival Guide</u>

Gingerbread Golem Recipes: Holiday Treats with a Magical Twist

The Infinite Key: Unlocking Mystical Secrets of the Ages

Enchanted Yule: A Wiccan and Pagan Guide to a Magical and Memorable Season

Dinosaurs of Power: Unlocking Ancient Magick

Astro-Dinos: The Cosmic Guide to Prehistoric Wisdom

Gallifrey's Yule Logs: A Festive Doctor Who Cookbook

The Dino Grimoire: Secrets of Prehistoric Magick

The Gift They Never Knew They Needed

The Gingerbread Golem's Culinary Alchemy: Enchanting Recipes for a Sweetly Dark Feast

A Time Lord Christmas: Holiday Adventures with the Doctor

Krampusproofing Your Home: Defensive Strategies for Yule

Silent Frights: A Collection of Christmas Creepypastas to Chill Your Bones

Santa Raptor's Jolly Carnage: A Dino-Claus Christmas Tale

Prehistoric Palettes: A Dino Wicca Coloring Journey

The Christmas Wishkeeper Chronicles

The Starlight Sleigh: A Holiday Journey

Elf Secrets: The True Magic of the North Pole

Reclaiming Time: How to Live More by Doing Less

Chronovore: The Eternal Nexus

The Mind Reset: Unlocking Your Inner Peace in a Chaotic World

Confidence Code: Building Unshakable Self-Belief

Baby the Vampire Terrier

Baby the Vampire Terrier's Christmas Adventure

Celestial Streams: The Content Creator's Astrology Manual

The Wealth Whisperer: Unlocking Abundance with Everyday Actions

The Energy Equation: Maximize Your Output Without Burning Out

The Happiness Algorithm: Science-Backed Steps to Joyful Living

Stress-Free Success: Achieving Goals Without Anxiety

Mindful Wealth: The New Blueprint for Financial Freedom

The Festive Flavors of New Year: A Culinary Celebration

The Master's Gambit: Keys of Eternal Power

Shadowed Secrets: Groundhog Day Mysteries

Beneath the Burrow: Lessons from the Groundhog

Spring's Whispers: The Groundhog's Prediction

The Limitless Mindset: Unlock Your Untapped Potential

The Focus Funnel: How to Cut Through Chaos and Get Results

Bold Moves: Building Courage to Live on Your Terms

The Daily Shift: Simple Practices for Lasting Transformation

The Quarter-Life Reset: Thriving in Your 20s and 30s

The Art of Shadowplay: Building Your Own Personal Myth

The Eternal Loop: Finding Purpose in Repetition

Burrowing Wisdom: Life Lessons from the Groundhog

Shadow Work: A Groundhog Day Perspective

Love in Bloom: 5-Minute Romantic Gestures

The Shadowspell Codex: Secrets of Forbidden Magick

The Burnout Cure: Finding Balance in a Busy World

The Groundhog Prophecy: Unlocking Seasonal Secrets

Nog Tales: The Spirited History of Eggnog

Winter's Wrath: The Complete Survival Blueprint for Extreme Freezes.

The Groundhog's Shadow: A Tale of Seasons
Burrowed Insights: Wisdom from the Groundhog
Sensual Strings: The Art of Erotic Bondage
Whispered Flames: Unlocking the Power of Fire Play
Forgotten Shadows: A Guide to Cryptids Lost to Time
Six Weeks of Secrets: Groundhog Day's Hidden Messages
Shadows and Cycles: Groundhog Day Reflections
The Art of Love Letters: Crafting the Perfect Message
Romantic Getaways at Home: Turning Your Space into Paradise
Purrfect Brews: A Cat Lover's Guide to Coffee and Companionship
The Groundhog's Wisdom: Timeless Lessons for Modern Life
The Shadow Oracle: Groundhog Day as a Predictor
Emerging from the Burrow: A Journey of Renewal
The Language of Love: Learning Your Partner's Love Style
Authorpreneur: The Ultimate Blueprint for Writing, Publishing, and Thriving as an Author
Weathering the Seasons: Groundhog Day Perspectives
Valentine's Day Magic: A Guide to Romantic Rituals
The Shadow Chronicles: Stories of Groundhog Day
Love and Laughter: Fun Games for Valentine's Day
AstroRealty: Unlocking the Stars for Property Success
The Groundhog's Path: A Guide to Seasonal Balance
Groundhog Day Diaries: Reflections in the Shadow
The Groundhog's Light: Illuminating the Path Ahead
Valentine's Traditions from Around the World
AI Wealth Revolution: Unlocking the Trillionaire Mindset
Love Rekindled: Reigniting Passion in Relationships
Single and Thriving: Self-Love on Valentine's Day
Emerald Legends: Mystical Tales of Ireland

Green Alchemy: Harnessing Nature's Magic

The Hearts of Horror: A Valentine's Day Nightmare

The Leprechaun's Guide to Wealth and Wisdom

Dancing with the Sidhe: Celebrating the Otherworld

Shamrocks and Shadows: Mysteries of the Green Isle

Emerald Energy: Harnessing Luck and Growth

The Gingerbread Golem's Valentine: A Sweetheart's Guide to Love and Enchantment

The Celtic Knot: Weaving Life and Destiny

Green Fire: Elemental Magic for St. Patrick's Day

Clover Chronicles: Finding Your Inner Luck

Ireland's Mystical Creatures: A Field Guide

Gingerbread Golem's Love Almanac

Prowl and Thrive: The Lion's Guide to Success

Love Alchemy: Transforming Your Life Through Heart Energy

WORLD DOMINATION: Woman's Rule 3:The New Life

The Midnight Rose: A Guide to Lunar Love Spells

The Forbidden Letters: Writing Your Own Love Prophecy

Luck and Lore: St. Patrick's Day for Modern Mystics

The Green Path: A Pagan Celebration of Renewal

The Dark Architect's Guide to Reprogramming Reality

Prankster's Paradise: A Guide to Harmless Hijinks

Manifest Your Reality: The Law of Attraction Simplified

The TARDIS Owner's Manual: Understanding the Doctor's Ship: *A complete guide to the TARDIS, its technology, secrets, and mysteries*

Starlit Romance: Astrology Secrets for Finding True Love

The Time Lord's Atlas: A Complete Guide to the Whoniverse: *A breakdown of the locations, planets, and dimensions explored in Doctor Who*

Sweetheart Shadows: The Dark Side of Love and Attraction

February Fire: Reigniting Passion in Every Area of Life

Timeless Love: Building and Maintaining Lasting Relationships

The Raven's Roar: Unlocking Unstoppable Confidence

Raven Sight: Awakening Intuition and Inner Wisdom

The Butterfly Effect: Small Changes, Big Transformations

Taming the Boogeyman: How to Conquer Your Inner Fears

The Magick of Green: Awakening Earth's Energy in You

The Entrepreneurial Mindset: Secrets to Business Success

The Hollowvale End

The Shadow Luck Ritual: Reclaiming Power from Your Dark Side

Spring Magick for Beginners: A Simple Guide to Seasonal Energy Work

Doctor Who: The Hollowvale Conundrum

The March of Miracles: Unlocking Synchronicities in Spring

Unveiling the Cosmos: A Guide to Stargazing and Space Exploration

The Ultimate Guide to Surviving an Economic Collapse

The AI Gold Rush: How to Profit from the AI Revolution

Bastet's Shadow: The Hidden Power of Feline Magick

The Bastet Codex: Unlocking the Goddess's Magickal Secrets

Purring Spells: Harnessing Bastet's Healing Frequencies

Bastet's Nine Lives: Rebirth, Transformation, and Immortality Spells

Primal Currents: Hydrocephalus Magick in the Path of Dino Wicca

The Digital Gold Rush: Mastering E-Commerce and Online Sales

Future Shock: Adapting to the Next Decade of Change

The Quantum Mindset: Think Like a Billionaire

Sacred Motherhood: Awakening the Divine Feminine Within

The Mother's Spellbook: Enchantments for Love, Protection, and Prosperity

The Witch's Guide to Parenting: Raising Empowered and Intuitive Children

The Magick of Motherhood: Reclaiming Your Power Through Rituals

The Pagan Path to Self-Love: A Goddess's Guide to Worth and Confidence

Wild Woman Magick: Unleashing Your Primal Power

The Money Magnet Blueprint: Unlocking Unlimited Wealth

Biohacking 101: Unlock Your Body's Full Potential

The Wild Father: A Pagan Guide to Strength and Wisdom

The Sacred Masculine: Unlocking Your Inner Power

The Druid's Compass

The Warrior's Mindset

The Father's Fire

Odin's Path

Ancestral Bonds

The House That Whispers

The Magician's Code

The Wild Hunt

The Green Man's Path

The Altar of Success

The Shadow and the Sword

The High Priestess's Guide to Energy Healing

The Lunar Mother

The Sacred Self-Care Grimoire

The Womb Wisdom Codex

The Wheel of the Mother

The Witch's Guide to Manifestation

The Q2 Reset

The Ultimate Guide to AI-Powered Passive Income

Escape the 9-5

AI Feline Fortunes

The Tear-Stained Grimoire

Razorblade Runes
Cemetery Sirens
The Midnight Wristwatch
The Town That Forgets
AI Horror & Creepypasta
The Hollow Frequency
The Breach Echo
The Quiet Between Worlds
The Sigil of Tharan-Khul
Summon the Vault of Y'ha'ten
The Becoming Codex
The Profit of Az'ra-nar
The Drowned Logos
Echoes of the Eldritch Will
The Deep Ledger
Necronomicon of Networth
Covenant of the Wealthwyrm
The Whisperer's Manifesto
The Rites of Azh-K'luth
The Ark of the Crawling Coin
The Tithe of Shadows
Inkheart Abyss
The Timewinds of Y'ha-nthlei
The Spiral Labyrinth of Azag-Nirrh
The Gallifreyan Heresy of the Black Pharaoh
The Psalms of Nyog-Sotha
Black Rain Alchemy
The Infinite Maw
The Entropic Blueprint
The Oracle of Sh'guul
The Book of Breach
The Drowned Saint's Testament
Dreamcraft of the Sleeper God

The Silence Market
Cthonomics: The Dark Wealth Algorithm
Invocation of the Ten-Eyed King
Wealthbound to the Wyrm Below
Become the Unnameable
Codex of the Sovereign Flame
Rituals of Relentless Becoming
The Shadow Ascends
The Eyes Beneath You
The Will That Wakes Worlds
Silence Is a Weapon
The Mirror That Screams
The Whisper Between Moments
The Mind That Devours Fear
The Myth of the Finished Self
The Architect of Your Madness
The Voice You've Buried
The Discipline of Madness
Stormborn: Awakening Your Inner Tempest
The Mind That Ate Time
Unbind Your Becoming
The Pact You Owe Yourself
The Devourer's Diet
The Acid That Carves the Path
The Tower You Must Burn
The Breath Between Worlds
Speak Like the Deep
The Labyrinth Within
The Spine of the Sea God
Rejection Is a Portal
The Crown You Refused
The Scar Is the Spell
The Lightless Flame

The Habit of Becoming Horrific
ChickenJockey Chaos
The Gatekeeper Within
You Are Not Your Name
The Compass of the Mad
The Archive of Unsent Letters
What the Mirror Can't Show You
The Knife You Needed
Worship Nothing, Become Everything
The Other Voice
The Body the World Forgot
The Vein of the Void
The Black Bone Codex
The Puzzle of the Hidden Self (Millennium Puzzle)
The Eye That Sees the Lie *(Millennium Eye)*
The Ring of Return (Millennium Ring)
The Rod of Relentless Will *(Millennium Rod)*
The Tally of the Soul (Millennium Tauk/Necklace)
The Key to the Locked Timeline (Millennium Key)
The Scale of Sacred Decisions (Millennium Scales)
Inferno Bites: The UnOfficial Minecraft Lava Cookbook
Rot in the Attic
Prana: The Hidden Force of Your Infinite Self
The Shadow Realm Within: Transforming Darkness Into Destiny
The Borderland Collapse
Claws of Protection: Bastet's Defensive Magick
Mr. Ring-a-Ding's Madness
Yugioh Astrology: Celestial Deckcraft and Duel Destiny (2026–2027 Edition)
The Seal You Signed: Unlocking the Power You Once Feared
The Puzzle of Infinite Minds: Unlocking the Mentalism Hidden Within

The Eye That Mirrors the All: Secrets of Inner Reflection
Doctor Who: The Toymaker's Broadcast
The Rod of Eternal Flow: Commanding the Currents of Vibration
Golden Eyes of Bastet: Enhancing Psychic Vision
The Key of Dual Forces: Balance Within the Polarity
The Scales of Living Rhythm: Timing the Dance of Life
The Necklace of Hidden Cause: Weaving the Webs of Fate
The Ring of Secret Masters: Rising Through the All Within All
Daggers of the Dying Deep
Bastet's Wealth and Fortune Magick: Prosperity Rituals of the Goddess
The Tide that Speaks
The Scrolls of Petosiris: 13 Rituals from the Feathered Eye
Petosiris and the Living Plague of Osirion
Feline Fire: Bastet's Passion and Love Magick
The Star Altar of Petosiris
Bastet's Whiskers: Supernatural Sensory Magick
The Bastet Grimoire
Feeding the Shadows
The Mouthless Prayer
The Spiral Wound
Becoming the Ibis: Lessons from Petosiris's Mind
The Crimson Coven: Cola Magick for Sweet Dominion
Sacred Cat's Paw
The Soda Zodiac: A Flavor for Every Sign
Covenant of the Crawling Flame
The Ink of Ish'Zur
Frothroot: The Thirst That Ate the World
The Golden Glyphs of Prosperity
The Etherbind Codex
Echoes of the Resistance: Reclaiming the You That Survived

Harnessed Minds: Breaking Free from Mental Control
The Eyes in the Smoke
Rootwake: The Carbon Covenant
Skitter Logic: Unlearning the Fear That Built You
Doctor Who: The World That Froths
Rootwake: The Fizz That Rewrites Flesh
Rootwake: Frothfather of the World
The Holly Pact: Blood Beneath the Mistletoe
The 2nd Mass Principle: Building Unbreakable Tribes
Web of Wits: A Survival Guide to Encounters with Anasi the Spider (Aunt Nancy)
The Hexbreaking Handbook: Effective Spells to Remove Curses
Pop Alchemy: Transform Your Life One Sip at a Time
The Mason Code: Leading in Unleadable Times
Petosiris and the Fifth Chamber of Thoth
The Ether Seed Within
The Parent of Tomorrow
Petosiris's Pyramid of Perpetual Wealth
Unlearn the World
Grimoire of the Hollow Tongue
Zodiac Weeds: Finding Your Strain Through the Stars
Aquarius Rises in the Bank
The Sugar God's Smile
The Skinclock Reversal: Biohacking the Face of Time
Debtburn: How to Obliterate What You Owe Forever

Get Some Tarot cards: https://www.makeplayingcards.com/sell/apophis-occult-shop

Get some shirts: https://www.bonfire.com/store/apophis-shirt-emporium/

<u>Instagrams:</u>
@apophis_enterprises,
@apophisbookemporium,
@apophisscardshop
Twitter: @apophisenterpr1
Tiktok:@apophisenterprise
Youtube: @sg1fan23477
Hive: @sg1fan23477
CheeLee: @SG1fan23477

Podcast: Apophis Chat Zone: https://open.spotify.com/show/5zXbrCLEV2xzCp8ybrfHsk?si=fb4d4fdbdce44dec

Newsletter: https://apophiss-newsletter-27c897.beehiiv.com/

If you want to support me or see posts of other projects that I have come over to: **buymeacoffee.com/mpetchinskg**
I post there daily several times a day

Get your Dinowicca or Christmas themed digital products, especially Santa Raptor songs and other musics. Here: **https://sg1fan23477.gumroad.com**

Apophis Yuletide Digital has not only digital Christmas items, but it will have all things with Dinowicca as well as other Digital products.